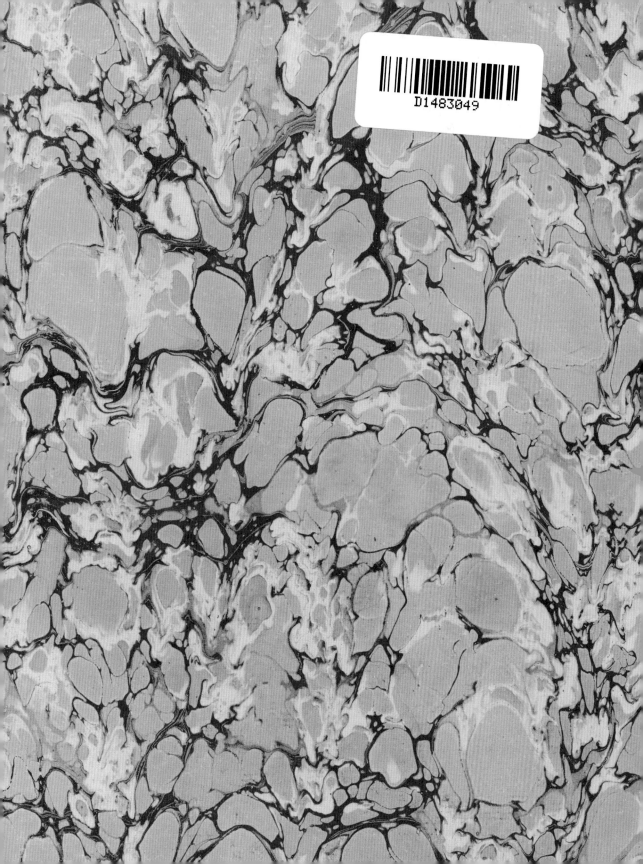

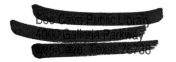

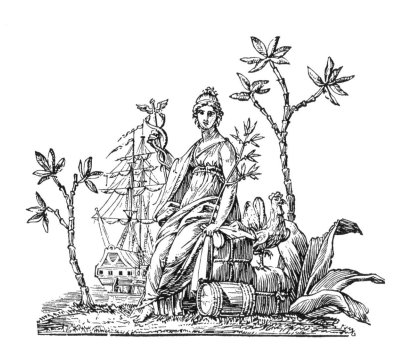

AN ATLAS

OF

NATURAL BEAUTY

BOTANICAL INGREDIENTS
FOR RETAINING AND ENHANCING BEAUTY

BY VICTOIRE DE TAILLAC AND RAMDANE TOUHAMI
FROM OFFICINE UNIVERSELLE BULY

SIMON & SCHUSTER

NEW YORK LONDON TORONTO SYDNEY NEW DELHI

Simon & Schuster
1230 Avenue of the Americas
New York, NY 10020

This publication contains the opinions
and ideas of its author. It is intended
to provide helpful and informative
material on the subjects addressed
in the publication. It is sold with the
understanding that the author and
publisher are not engaged in rendering
medical, health, or any other kind
of personal professional services in
the book. The reader should consult
his or her medical, health, or other
competent professional before adopting
any of the suggestions in this book or
drawing inferences from it. The author
and publisher specifically disclaim all
responsibility for any liability, loss, or risk,
personal or otherwise, which is incurred
as a consequence, directly or indirectly,
of the use and application of any of the
contents of this book.

First Simon & Schuster hardcover edition
November 2018
Originally published in Great Britain in
2017 by Ebury Press

SIMON & SCHUSTER and colophon
are registered trademarks of Simon &
Schuster, Inc.

For information about special discounts for
bulk purchases, please contact Simon &
Schuster Special Sales at 1-866-506-1949
or business@simonandschuster.com.

The Simon & Schuster Speakers Bureau
can bring authors to your live event. For
more information or to book an event
contact the Simon & Schuster Speakers
Bureau at 1-866-248-3049 or visit our
website at www.simonspeakers.com.

Manufactured in the United States of
America

10   9   8   7   6   5   4   3   2   1

Library of Congress Cataloguing-in-
Publication Data is available

ISBN 978-1-5011-9735-2
ISBN 978-1-5011-9736-9 (ebook)

SUMMARY

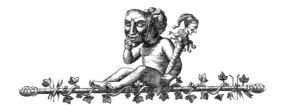

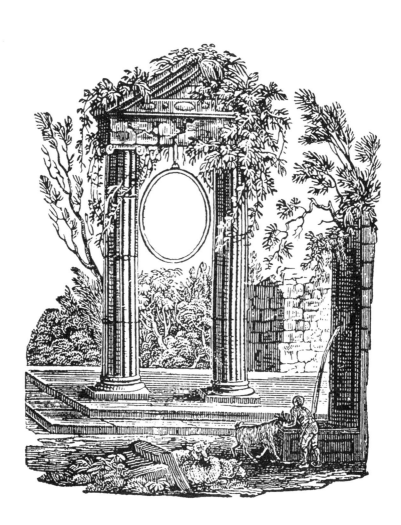

NATURAL BEAUTY

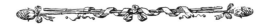

Nothing is simpler, more enjoyable, more self-evident, or more efficient than taking good, natural care of yourself. Nothing is easier than devoting the requisite amount of time to it—no more than you would spend on commercial cosmetics—and nothing is more pleasant than giving meaning to your beauty rituals. Just like a short breather, this can fit into any day's schedule. It is a lifestyle which does not require much space and does not even involve fancy words or overly intricate steps—a source of delight that lends sweetness to everyday life.

And that must be the world's best-kept beauty secret: there is no need to go overboard to stay at the top of your game. All it takes are a few gentle movements and the many things nature and nurture have to offer, generously and often economically.

This book also provides the perfect opportunity to regain control: it is no longer about brands, fads, and appearances—it is about you. The simple knowledge we have gathered here, along with your own experimentations, should give you the gratifying ability and privilege to care for yourself and your loved ones.

Beauty is not all about marketing and promises. To attain beauty and well-being you must keep it simple and speak the truth. This type of natural beauty exists, and it is within reach. Discovering these authentic beauty secrets also provides an opportunity to travel through time and space, to marvel at the riches of the plant world and at man's ingenuity in discovering and making the most of them. Nature-based beauty has the precious added benefit of encouraging us to use gentle organic ingredients, whose active concentration is much greater than that of the average industrial product. With these beauty recipes and natural products, which L'Officine Universelle has had the pleasure of collecting and sharing, you know exactly what your skin is getting: nothing but the best.

At L'Officine Universelle Buly, we select with passion and curiosity the very best of these "raw" materials. By favoring traditional agriculture and the work of rural cooperatives, we support the endurance and growth of these communities, which are rightly proud of their know-how and of perpetuating these traditions.

This book lists eighty ingredients and raw materials to take good care of yourself, along with tested recipes garnered from the collective experience of all of the world's cultures. These simple and precious products have been kept alive by continued use and by the beauty habits of the inhabitants of all continents.

This is an experience that is simultaneously millennial and yet ever so contemporary.

Time stops, beauty is universal. Re-enchant your bathroom, join in the game, and create your own beneficial and efficient rituals.

FIRST THINGS FIRST

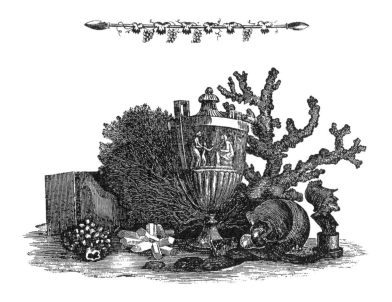

Don't be fazed by raw materials: you will soon feel at home with their striking simplicity, which will fuel your experience, your knowledge, and your creativity as you unlock their benefits.

Just as we do, make sure to select the purest, most naturally active ingredients: be exacting about their quality, their source (whether organic or classic), and their freshness. And each time you try a new ingredient, take the time to test it beforehand on the crook of your elbow, to make sure it does not trigger any allergy or irritation.

The hygiene of your hands, cloths, tools, and various containers must also be impeccable. Sterilizing jars is a simple and indispensable step: your creations will then keep for anywhere between a day and several months, depending on their nature and shelf life. Remember that water is a veritable breeding ground for certain bacteria, which is not the case for oils. Trust your judgment, your nose, and your eyes. If in doubt, don't use (or stop using) your creations completely.

The properties, indications, and usage instructions for all the active ingredients in this book draw on our experience in the realm of cosmetics, but also on reference books and from canvassing beauty rituals and traditions from all over the world. Nonetheless, this information is intended as a guide only; in no way does it constitute medical information, nor can we be held responsible for it. For any therapeutic usage of the essential oils, hydrolates, and plants or plant powders mentioned herein, make sure to consult a doctor first.

THE RIGHT RITUALS

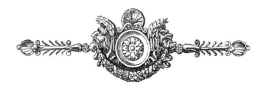

REMOVING MAKEUP

○

Returning to your natural state before bed
is an indispensable ritual. The skin must
be thoroughly and gently rid of all makeup,
and with it the day's many trials. Indeed,
whatever your skin type, skin is fragile and
must be allowed to breathe. A makeup
removal solution should be very simple:
just a touch of floral water and a few drops
of natural oil sprinkled on a cotton pad—
as many times as necessary to remove all
traces of makeup or urban grime.

CLEANSING THE FACE

○

The feeling of a clean face is one of life's
simplest pleasures, but this step should
be handled carefully. Washing is good—
stripping is not. You must find the ritual
that will leave you fresh and satisfied,
without upsetting the balance of your
skin. Perhaps some warm, clear water—
whether mineral or filtered—or a little
floral water on a cotton pad? Using soap is
unnecessary! So is rubbing the skin, which
tends to dry it. Overly aggressive cleansing
will tire, irritate, and inflame the skin.

CLEANSING THE HAIR

○

This may sound simple, and yet! Our
obsession with shampoo, which we
insist on lathering on frenetically, and
which we rinse off hastily, goes against
our objectives. . . . The art of proper
hair cleaning means a hair-embellishing
treatment: select an organic, gentle
shampoo, start by dispensing the desired
dosage into a bowl and diluting it with
some tepid water, pour it onto your damp
hair, and gently and slowly massage with
the tips of your fingers until clean. Then
rinse, rinse, rinse . . . and to complete the
rinsing process, you may want to try some
diluted hair care vinegar, which imparts
shine and removes the last remaining
impurities. Ideally, little by little you
should try to space out each time you use
shampoo, first by one day, and then two.
The scalp will then learn to recover its
balance on its own.

SCRUBBING

○

The skin is all about touch. Sometimes,
just by running your fingers over it, you

may feel the need to refine its grain, to soften it. Obviously, the thin skin of the face requires a greater level of care and gentleness than that of the body, which is often less fragile. But it is just as obvious that neither should be constantly worn down, letting the skin balance itself. Rather, remember to exfoliate your body once a week, and give your face a rest — a gentle scrub once every ten days will suffice.

MASSAGING THE FACE

o

A facial massage could become a daily pleasure, whenever you apply a cleansing milk, a plant oil, or a cream. It should be done from the center out. Circular motions, tiny pinches . . . it is the simplest of royal treatments for the face, which helps to maintain or recover radiance: it relaxes and smoothes the facial features, all the while oxygenating and calming the skin.

MASSAGING THE BODY

o

Self-massages, whether dry or wet (in a warm bath or shower), are a good way to unknot tense muscles and to make a fresh start. Your body could benefit from special treatment with a regularly applied beneficial oil, and from a short, focused massage as you apply your everyday cream.

BRUSHING THE BODY

o

Whether in the shower or in a dry setting, rubbing yourself from top to toe, using a brush with relatively firm bristles, will bring the skin tremendous vitality, improve

its appearance, ward off fat dimples, and soften it without damaging it. What could be better? This treatment can be performed daily.

BRUSHING THE HAIR

o

The myth about giving your hair one hundred brush strokes a day has a romantic ring to it, but not all heads of hair require the same rituals, and it would be disastrous for some. . . . Gently brushing or combing your hair rids it of impurities, makes it shinier, and stimulates the scalp. It is important to find the right tool for you, which should be high-quality and suited to your hair so as not to damage it. The proper pace at which to brush depends on you and on whether you like your hair coiffed or disheveled.

MASKS

o

If you're taking the time to apply a mask, chances are you can also set aside five minutes to concoct it yourself. A little clay and vegetable powder, some floral water, and natural or essential oil, and there you have it: a highly natural and efficient treatment for the face or hair! Each mask is an opportunity for your body and mind to catch their breath: such attentions will also boost your morale.

THE RIGHT PREPARATIONS

TO THE BATH WITH YOU!

Steam baths, foot baths, and full-body baths are natural beauty treatments that are as simple as they are thrilling. Hydrolates, diluted essential oils, pesticide-free botanicals, clays—these ingredients will enrich this beneficial ritual and efficiently improve your radiance and well-being.

MASKS AND POULTICES

Nothing could be simpler or more beneficial than preparing an on-the-spot mask, which will be more naturally efficient than most commercial cosmetic products. A spoonful of powder, a few drops of oil (whether natural or essential), a little floral water in the palm of your hand or in a bowl, and there you have it: a treatment that is perfectly suited to the needs of your skin and hair, and to the current climate!

DRYING

In order to dry plants, one must tie them together in a bunch and hang them, inflorescences or leaves toward the ground, in a dry and well-ventilated room. To make this effective and avoid the onset of mold, it's important they dry quickly. Dried plants can be kept in tightly shut jars for up to a year—be sure to label them with the name of the plant and the date on which they were dried.

INFUSIONS

Infusions are a quick and simple way to extract the properties of the plants' more fragile parts—the leaves, flowers, and stems. For every cup of water (whether mineral or filtered), use one spoonful of dried plant material or two spoonfuls of freshly cut plant. Bring the water to a simmer and, while you wait, place the plant you would like to infuse at the bottom of a teapot. Pour the simmering water over the plant and promptly close the lid. Simmering water, as opposed to boiling water, does not "burn" the plants; neither does it obliterate their active ingredients. Allow to infuse for about ten minutes. Once it has cooled down, this infusion can be used as rinsing water for the hair or as a facial lotion.

DECOCTIONS
○

A decoction is hardly more complex to prepare than an infusion. It is simply a more "robust" method of extracting the active ingredients from the tougher parts of the plants: seeds, roots, barks, etc. For every cup of water (whether mineral or filtered), use one spoonful of dried plant material or two spoonfuls of freshly cut plant. Be sure to dice the plant into tiny pieces so as to facilitate the extraction. Place the plants in a saucepan (preferably one that is made out of glass), cover with water, and bring to a medium boil. Boil the botanicals for about ten minutes before turning off the heat. Though it is more concentrated than an infusion, a decoction can be used in the same way.

MACERATES
○

Macerates are easier to prepare using dried plants. Whether they are fresh or dry, the botanicals must be diced into tiny pieces and then plunged into the neutral oil of your choice—preferably one that is odorless and keeps well, such as grapeseed oil. Allow to macerate for one to two weeks under direct sunlight, before filtering the macerate using a cheesecloth, pressing down on the plants so as to maximize the resulting active concentration. A macerate will keep for up to six months in a vial stored in a cool, dry place and away from sunlight.

BAIN-MARIE
○

A bain-marie is a simple cooking technique in which the heating vessel itself is immersed halfway in a "bath" of simmering water. This will prevent the plants and other ingredients from being brought to an excessive temperature, which would negatively affect the shelf life and the integrity of the ointments you are preparing.

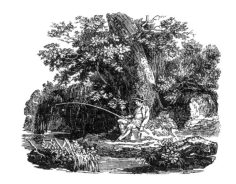

THE RIGHT TOOLS

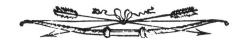

The hand is guided by the tool's perfection. A few well-executed motions and well-chosen instruments are just as effective as a whole lot of overly complicated beauty formulations. We encourage you to acquire the best and most durable ones and to make regular use of them. They will prove useful to carry out, quickly and effectively, the rituals and recipes collected in this book. The list that follows is not exhaustive. It itemizes those which have seemed indispensable to us. Perfection, comfort, the handle and material of the implement . . . everything is conducive to good use and regular practice. What is beautiful is also usually pleasant to use.

METAL BOWL

◉

This indestructible, heavy-duty, and well-proportioned bowl fits in the hand; it can slip into the bathtub and float on the bathwater. It is an essential ally for making the perfect mixture, diluting a shampoo, or collecting and distributing a rinsing water.

CERAMIC OR GLASS BOWL

◉

Indispensable for those ingredients that metal can damage through oxidation (clays, for the most part).

BAMBOO WHISK

◉

Neutral and allows for a fine emulsion. It must be properly rinsed and dried after each use. In Japan, it is most commonly used to emulsify matcha—powdered green tea.

CONTAINERS FOR YOUR CREATIONS

◉

Beauty and function can go hand in hand: a small glass jar with a dropper, a small glass bottle. . . .

HAIRBRUSH

◉

It is all about finding the model, the bristle strength, and the handle that will be best suited to your hair. After each brushing, your brush must be rid of any hair that has accumulated. At regular intervals, it must be dusted using a tough scrubbing brush which is to be run between the rows of bristles.

FINE- AND LARGE-TOOTHED COMBS

◉

There are as many types of comb as there are types of hair and usages. Pick whichever is best suited to you.

SUPPLE NAIL BRUSH

◦

Nail brushing should be performed daily. A supple brush, both firm and soft, is the indispensable accessory for hand and foot cleansing.

MAKEUP BRUSHES

◦

A good makeup brush must always be properly cleaned with water and soap, properly rinsed, and properly dried; it offers the best and surest way to apply a mask to the face or hair.

BODY BRUSH

◦

Whether fitted with a handle or a strap, it can be as tough or as soft as you wish. Some will like it as simple as it gets; others will prefer more sophisticated models equipped with copper bristles for deeper drainage. In this case, the brush should be kept dry.

NATURAL SPONGE

◦

Nothing is healthier, simpler, or more pleasantly efficient than a genuine natural sponge—to complete the removal of makeup or of a mask, or simply for showering or bathing. . . . Well-rinsed and left to dry in the open air, a high-quality natural sponge will last for years.

FINE COTTON GAUZE

◦

To create your own "sachets" (see pages 254–5), infuse certain botanicals, or hold certain masks, cotton gauze is a classic that you can buy in the form of bandages at any pharmacy.

TOWELS

◦

Depending on how finely it is woven, on the material it is made of, and on its thickness, a towel can absorb quickly or slowly; it can gently exfoliate the skin or vigorously activate circulation. In addition to the classic terry cloth, it is recommended to have drier types of cloth on hand—honeycomb towels, for instance.

TUB

◦

Whether it is made of enameled metal or plastic, a wide, capacious tub is ideal for footbaths and nail care.

MAKEUP-REMOVING COTTON PADS

◦

Natural cotton—less whitened or treated than synthetic types—should be used for gentler beauty treatments.

FROM THE KITCHEN TO THE BATHROOM

◦

For crushing and mixing botanicals, a good grinder and a mortar and pestle should follow you from the kitchen into the bathroom.

TABLE
OF
INGREDIENTS

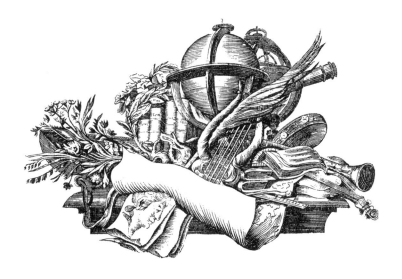

20

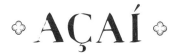

✣ AÇAÍ ✣

Oil (berries) — Origin: Amazonia

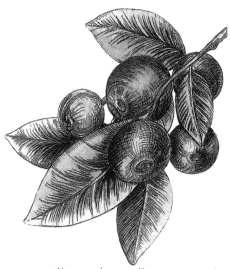

Euterpe oleracea, Euterpe precatoria

THE AMAZON'S GOLD

○

In Amazonia, there are two types of açaí: *açaí-do-Pará*, *Euterpe oleracea*, a palm tree from East Amazonia, and *açaí-do-mato*, *Euterpe precatoria*, from Central Amazonia. Both grow in hot, humid climates; they thrive best in marshland and help maintain the equilibrium of their natural habitat, namely the forests that line the Amazon River. Keep in mind that the palm tree is a type of grass, albeit a giant one, rather than an actual "tree." Each infructescence — or cluster — has a few hundred fruits at its top, which take on a deep violet hue when ripe. The açaí's purple berry boasts potent benefits: it is a godsend for the rural populations that cultivate it.

TEACHINGS FROM TIME IMMEMORIAL

○

The açaí's properties were already celebrated by pre-Columbian civilizations, which made abundant use of it: its roots, administered as a decoction, treated jaundice and malaria; its fruit alleviated skin conditions; and its seeds were reputed to bring down fevers. Açaí wine was one of the pillars of these societies' diets. Thanks to the fruit's high concentration of antioxidants — ten times that of black grapes — and its protein content, which equals that of an egg, it is now highly prized by proponents of alternative organic and vegan diets.

In the 1990s, the fruit's popularity spread to Rio, where it can now be enjoyed in açaí bars in the form of ice cream or granola. Its success and worldwide exportation feed a profitable market and foster the development of plantations. Recently, açaí has become an expensive commodity for the Ribeirinhos, the people of the river, who have relied on it for centuries.

THE CRYING FRUIT

○

Içà-çai is featured in a tragic legend that tells of the immense sorrow of a young woman who, during a particularly severe period of famine for her people, witnessed the sacrifice of her infant daughter and

> *"It is better to grow green again
> than to always be green."*

MADAME DE SÉVIGNÉ

died at the foot of the fruit-covered tree
that was to save her people from hunger.

ON COLLECTING AÇAÍ OIL

Just as rich as it is hard, this precious
fruit is 90% seed and 10% pulp. It must be
harvested with great care and picked by
hand. Pickers have no choice but to climb
up the palm tree's stem — in dry weather so
as not to slip. The berries are then cold-
pressed. Their densely textured oil is dark
and green, much like the primal forest.
It oozes a naturally pungent scent, which
fades quickly after application.

THE BENEFITS

Spectacularly efficient after a few days' use,
açaí oil helps prevent the skin from drying
out and the passage of time from leaving
its marks. It is made up of more than 50%
oleic acid (omega-9), which improves the
skin's elasticity and contributes to its
optimal hydration. High in tannins,
it has anti-inflammatory, antioxidant,
and astringent properties that make
it the best ally of combination as well as
dry skin types. Its high concentration of
vitamin F protects the cells and fosters
their turnover.

JUST A FEW DROPS

Desperate situations call for drastic
remedies: açaí oil is the choice elixir of
distressed skin. It is highly effective on
skin that has been weakened by extreme
levels of fatigue, by exposure to high winds
and harsh sunlight, or on skin that displays
signs of aging. Its smell is a bit too pungent
to be applied in the morning, and its green
tinge fades after application. Two or three
drops of açaí oil, massaged on a freshly
cleansed face every night at bedtime,
work wonders! The skin becomes softer,
stronger, and more supple. It is refreshed
and recovers its firmness.

AÇAÍ OIL–BASED RECIPES
from Officine Universelle

HELP — LIFESAVING MASK FOR SKIN IN NEED

Listen to your epidermis: sight and touch should guide your cosmetic instincts. Tight skin and a dull complexion call for immediate action.

Dilute a teaspoon of açaí powder in two spoonfuls of honey; then gently incorporate the blended pulp of half an avocado. Those with very dry skin can add three drops of açaí oil to this mixture. Put on your bathrobe, clear any loose hair strands away from your face, and apply this supple, bright green mask by hand. Get comfortably settled and leave on for twenty minutes. Rinse carefully and pat dry.

Abracadabra, your skin is now smoothed and soothed; now, don't forget to drink plenty of water or herbal tea.

MAKEUP REMOVER FOR ALL OCCASIONS

Your skin has endured all your cosmetic experiments — but has it upped its tolerance threshold? Daily makeup removal using açaí oil should be your go-to method, instead of becoming more and more demoralized as you wait for better skin days.

For a very gentle facial cleanse, apply two or three drops of açaí oil to a cotton pad sprinkled — but never soaked! — with rose water. Run the pad gently over the whole face and neckline in small circular motions without ever actually rubbing the skin. It is recommended not to rinse, nor to leave to air-dry, but rather to pat the face and neck with a fine, clean, dry cloth.

An ideal cleanse that leaves your skin immaculate and soothed.

SPECIAL SERUM FOR SPLIT ENDS

Having fallen victim to the "blond princess syndrome," and despite all sound advice, you refuse to cut your brown hair and wear your split ends proudly. Come to your senses and care for your hair with açaí oil.

Several times a week, apply two drops of açaí oil and one drop of hemp oil — gently warmed and mixed between your palms — onto the bottom third of your hair, brushed or unbrushed, depending on the intended effect: this combination efficiently heals split ends and protects the hair from further damage.

✦ ALOE VERA ✦

Oily macerate, gel (leaves) — Origin: North Africa

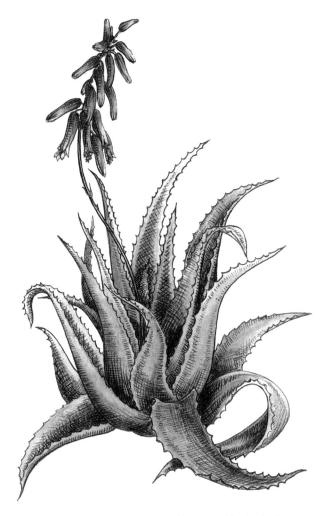

Aloe vera, Aloe barbadensis

A RIVER RUNS THROUGH IT

◦

Famed for its cosmetic and medicinal uses, aloe vera is a succulent from the Liliaceae family. Nicknamed "the desert lily," this aloe is known for its long, smooth, and fleshy leaves fringed with very tough thorns. It grows under the fire of the sun on dry terrain, and the wind and stones are the only nourishment it needs. Within its thick leaves lies an abundant pulp, as transparent and fresh as a gel, a miraculous source.

TEACHINGS FROM TIME IMMEMORIAL

○

The origins of aloe vera remain murky for botanists. The plant reportedly originates from either the Arabian Peninsula or North Africa. Its name derives from the Arabic word *alloeh*, meaning "bitter," and from the Latin word *vera*, meaning "true." Its use and prescription have been documented in all Middle Eastern cultures. In the case of the Sumerians, in the 3rd millennium BC, clay tablets testify to its therapeutic benefits. The Egyptians considered aloe vera to be a longevity elixir, and it is mentioned several times in the Ebers Papyrus—named after its translator—which dates back to the 16th century BC, and contains the famed *Book on the Preparation of Medicine for All Parts of the Human Body*. It celebrates the impressive healing power of aloe in embellishing, stimulating, and caring for the skin, as well as warding off hair loss.

ON COLLECTING ALOE VERA

○

At full maturity, aloe leaves contain an almost transparent and viscous mucilaginous gel, which is harvested with an expert cut so as to preserve both the plant and its pulp. This gel can be applied directly onto the skin, but it oxidizes very quickly. For better preservation, incised leaves were once hung from the tip to let the juice flow out slowly, before cooking reduced it to a syrup. A more recent method opts for crushing and pulverizing the leaves. The powder that is thus obtained is highly stable and easy to preserve; it is used in many aloe vera–based products. This precious gel is nowadays also harvested by extraction, and pasteurization has finally made it possible to package fresh aloe vera juice. Macerating the plant in a neutral vegetable oil—such as sunflower or jojoba—is another way to harness its properties and to convey them as simply as possible to the skin. If there is some aloe vera in your garden, this source of freshness is within arm's reach! Exercising just a little caution, it is not that hard to harvest some of its gel. Just cut one fine leaf at the base, choose a slice, cut off its spiny sides, run it under fresh water, and let the gel flow onto your skin.

THE BENEFITS

○

Aloe vera extract is rich in vitamin A, which increases cell turnover and alleviates dark spots; in vitamin C, which stimulates microcirculation within the skin; and in vitamins B and E, which help the cells fight oxidative stress. Its high concentration of minerals, trace elements, and eighteen amino acids explain the potency of its effects on the skin and the accuracy of its nickname in traditional Chinese medicine, where it is known as the "harmonious remedy." It is particularly effective when it comes to soothing the discomfort of sunburn and to revitalizing damaged and parched skin. It works wonders on skin that lacks vitality, which it smoothes and revives.

JUST A FEW DROPS

The joys of life as a couple, still passionate on a day-to-day basis, entail some embarrassing or irritating side effects. Have fiery kisses from a three-day beard left marks on your delicate cheeks? Two pats of aloe vera gel, a few minutes before stepping out the door of your love nest, and you'll be back to your old self—others will be none the wiser! Highly effective on a face that has been dried out by the open air and nothing short of miraculous on hands after gardening or indulging in DIY projects, a pat of aloe vera gel on freshly cleansed skin will be a fit reward for any exertion.

"Four plants are indispensable to man's well-being: wheat, grapes, olives, and Aloe. The first one nourishes him, the second allows his spirit to rise, the third brings him harmony, and the fourth heals him."

CHRISTOPHER COLUMBUS

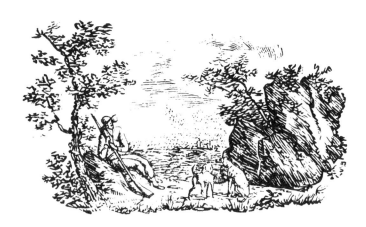

ALOE VERA–BASED RECIPES

from Officine Universelle

SOS SUN BALM

You knew better, but you couldn't resist the urge to be in communion with our neighboring star and the hot sand. . . . The deed is done, but the remedy may be within arm's reach.

Don't hesitate to apply a generous, healthy dollop of aloe vera gel to sunburn—the cooling and soothing effect is immediate. Once calm has been restored, restorative sleep once again becomes possible.

Remember, in a passionate relationship with the sun, the only choice is moderation. "Too much" is not an option! Traveling around with a tube of aloe vera gel does not exempt you from regularly ducking under the shade of a tree or a parasol!

SERUM TO SMOOTH OUT EYE BAGS

Sometimes, you wish your eyes would speak less of the passage of time and how tired you are. The area surrounding the eyes is often in crisis: the skin is dry, thin, sensitive. . . . Add the collective benefits of the three ingredients in this serum to one delicious coffee, and there you are, ready to look your Monday morning straight in the eye.

Using a whisk, emulsify two tablespoons of aloe vera gel, one teaspoon of cornflower

hydrolate, and three drops of tamanu oil. Keep the mixture in the fridge in a little vial or a roll-on for up to a week. Apply on the area around the eyes every morning when you wake. Gently rub until it is absorbed, and your gaze will be at its finest.

ANTI–HAIR LOSS HYDRATING MASK

The injustice of hair loss is a depressing form of capillary trauma. . . . Lay off the pixie dust and instead, invest in the ideal brush or comb. Enhance your scalp massages with a weekly treatment, to be performed in the quiet of your bathroom and combined with the scent of your favorite candle, the reading of a beloved poem, and the joyous sight of your hair recovering its radiance.

Thoroughly mix two tablespoons of aloe vera macerate, one tablespoon of coconut milk, and two or three drops of ginger essential oil using a small bamboo whisk. Apply this mask to the roots of dry hair, massaging it for two minutes, and finish by applying it all the way to the tips. Leave on for about twenty minutes, then wash out with a very gentle shampoo.

✦ ALUM STONE ✦

Stone and powder — Origin: Syria

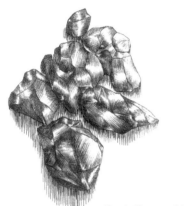

Aluminiferous schist

PURITY STONE

In its natural state, this veined, translucent, and rather brittle rock is made up of sulfuric acid, aluminum oxide, and potassium sulfate. Historical evidence suggests that alunite mines were first exploited in Syria and Egypt, where the rocks come right up to the surface, as they do in some parts of Europe, notably Bohemia and Saxony.

TEACHINGS
FROM TIME IMMEMORIAL

The ancient Greek philosopher and alchemist Theophrastus published a work entitled "On salt, niter and alum." Indeed, alum is a close relative of the famed natron, which was used in medicine and for embalming bodies throughout ancient Egypt. In the Middle Ages, this stone was used to stabilize dyes and pigments. Naturally astringent and antiseptic, it is the traditional aftershave treatment of barbers. To clarify and purify water, one can throw some alum into it — it is reputed to remove impurities. In the Maghreb, mouth ulcers and other oral ailments are healed by gargling some pure water enhanced with alum powder. In Morocco, the so-called Roman's mixture, which contains alum powder, jujube, and coarse salt, is said to ward off the evil eye.

ON COLLECTING ALUM STONE

Traditionally, alum stone is divided, cut, and polished by hand into a soft, smooth cobble, which can be easily run over the skin of the cheeks, neck, and chin. There are two types of alum stone — the natural version, which is preferable, and one synthesized from crystallized alunite. Natural alum stone is translucent, veined, and ribbed. By contrast, the reconstituted stone is opaque and homogenous.

THE BENEFITS

The aluminum sulfate and potassium sulfate that are naturally present in alum stone have antibacterial and astringent properties that help tighten the skin's pores, minimize sweating, and encourage hemostasis after the occurrence of minor cuts.

JUST A FEW DROPS

In order to enjoy the full benefits of alum stone, it is best to opt for the natural version. To use, briefly douse the alum stone with fresh water and apply to damp skin. It is an ideal aftershave which prevents the onset of ingrown hairs and blemishes. It is also a natural alternative to deodorants, as it minimizes sweating and inhibits the growth of bacteria. In powder form it can also be used as talcum powder, or as a bath salt, to treat clammy hands and feet.

ALUM-BASED RECIPES

from Officine Universelle

SOS ALUM BATH

A hand and foot bath to promote clarity and heal minor aches.

Is your skin cut and scraped? To calm the damage wrought by gardening and to purify the skin, relieve ingrown nails before a pedicure, or cleanse the wound on your knee after a fall, allow a heaping tablespoon of alum stone powder to dissolve in a small tub filled with warm water. Soak your hands or feet in it for about ten minutes, or douse the area that needs to be cleaned, and rinse with clear water. After this treatment, which you can supplement with some lemon if your nails are stained, gently massage half a teaspoon of shea butter onto work-weary hands and around the nails.

PURIFYING HAND AND FOOT SCRUB

Sandal alert! Feet that are fresh out of winter or too calloused for summer can be beautified with this weekly scrub.

In a small bowl, carefully mix one level tablespoon of alum stone powder with two teaspoons of argan oil and two drops of geranium essential oil. Gently scrub the feet—their soles, heels, and toes—with this mixture, which, by the way, can also be used as a hand scrub. Finish on the back of your hands and rinse with warm water.

"Only stone is innocent."

HEGEL

❖ AMLA ❖

Powder (fruit) — Origin: India

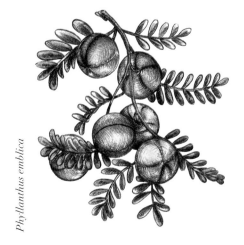

Phyllanthus emblica

THE PRINCESS AND THE PEA

◦

Known as *amalaki* in Sanskrit and nicknamed the "longevity tree," this shrub thrives in the humid forests of Northern India, Nepal, and Sri Lanka. It is grown with great care for its fruit — a sort of precious gooseberry — and is in fact positively "pampered": in summer, farmers protect its trunk from the sun with a layer of mud, and light small fires around it whenever the temperature drops dramatically in order to keep its leaves from falling. . . .

TEACHINGS FROM TIME IMMEMORIAL

◦

The saying goes that amla is to plants as gold is to rocks: popular wisdom recommends sitting beneath an amalaki tree to stimulate vitality and health. Rich in vitamins, it is one of the constituents of *triphala*, an Indian Ayurvedic panacea and one of the oldest Ayurvedic healing formulae, reputed to balance the organs and alleviate their ailments. This Indian gooseberry is famous for its tremendous antiaging powers: it is reportedly the great secret behind the long-lasting youthfulness of Indian ladies and their splendid jet-black hair.

ON COLLECTING AMLA

◦

In the northern hemisphere, its fruits are harvested in December and January. With their vivid, bright green color and their sourness, they can be eaten raw or dried, stewed into jellies, or preserved as jams or syrups. For cosmetic use, the berries are dried in the open air and later crushed to a powder to be used as a natural dye.

THE BENEFITS

◦

Amla's reputation is for its high concentration of vitamins: Vitamins A and C foster cell turnover in the epidermis. Vitamin C stimulates microcirculation within the skin. Vitamin E protects skin and hair from oxidation. Amla's beneficial, fortifying, and invigorating effects derive from its high concentration of polyphenols: tannins, flavonoids, gallic acid, and ellagic acid.

A FEW PINCHES

Amla is the plant that Indian women use most often to care for their sumptuous hair. Its powder is mixed with a vegetable oil to enhance and soften the hair, stimulate its growth, and ward off the onset of grayness. It also tints the hair, and so is best suited to brunettes.

AMLA-BASED RECIPES

from Officine Universelle

STIMULATING AND NOURISHING PRE-SHAMPOO FLUID FOR DARK HAIR

One can enjoy the passage of time and still try to postpone its effects: this formula preserves the vigor of brown hair and delays the onset of grayness.

In a large jar, mix ¾ cup plus 1 tablespoon of coconut oil with 1¾ ounces of amla powder. Let it rest for a week, shaking the jar daily, so that a fine maceration can take place. Apply a small amount of this fluid to dry hair, section by section, and leave on for at least ten minutes prior to shampooing. This potent mixture keeps for a month in a closed jar, away from direct sunlight.

FAST-GROWTH HAIR FORTIFIER

Think of this rinsing treatment as a journey, which cosmetic explorers will relish.

Boil ten or so amla berries (after removing the seeds), or a tablespoon of powder, in two cups of filtered water. Once the fruit has softened, add six fresh, neutral henna leaves and remove from the heat. Cover and allow to infuse until the water cools down. Filter and store the amla water in a bottle, which you should keep in a cool place. To stimulate hair growth, use to rinse your hair after each gentle shampoo.

⬧ ANDIROBA ⬧

Oil (seeds) — Origin: Brazil

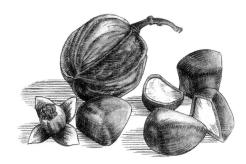

Carapa guianensis

JUNGLE POWER

❂

In the springtime, *Carapa guianensis* is covered with attractive, sweet-scented red flowers. It is a tropical tree that thrives in the Amazon rain forest and Central America, on the land lining the river that snakes through the forest. The andiroba grows in the vicinity of the rubber tree and the ucuhuba, or baboonwood. Its fruit, shaped like a tiny flying saucer, contains about ten nuts.

TEACHINGS FROM TIME IMMEMORIAL

❂

This tree has been revered since ancient times by the peoples of the Amazon rain forest. The Indians of the warlike Munduruku tribe used andiroba oil to mummify their spoils of war. The leaves of the andiroba, very bitter to the taste, were among the ingredients of concoctions used to cure fevers and digestive disorders. For centuries people have been extracting a rich, light oil from its nuts, and praises have been sung about its rejuvenating power. The andiroba contains substances that repel insects and parasites, notably head lice and ticks. It also gently soothes bites and stings. The Brazilian health department has entered *Carapa guianensis* into the country's national registry of useful medicinal plants.

ON COLLECTING ANDIROBA OIL

❂

In the delta of the Amazon River, the natives used to pick up andiroba fruit that had washed off onto the river's banks and bends and boil them in water for several hours. Dried in the shade for several days and then shelled, the fruit was simply sliced and packed together in a punctured container, letting its precious brown oil flow out slowly through the holes. This traditional, almost ritualistic mode of collection is no longer in use. Nowadays, the fruit is harvested differently and the oil obtained by cold-pressing. It is characterized by a pale yellow tint and a slight opacity. Though it remains fluid in warm climates, this thin-textured substance hardens as soon as the temperature drops below 77°F. All you have to do then is to run the vial under warm water before use.

THE BENEFITS

Oleic acid—omega-9—and palmitic acid, of which andiroba oil has a high concentration, are two fatty acids that help with hydrating and softening the skin. Phytosterols stimulate microcirculation and improve the complexion. Andirobin and vitamin F, thanks to their antiseptic and soothing properties, are a veritable balm for "teenage," damaged skin, as well as skin marked by blemishes or acne.

JUST A FEW DROPS

Perplexed by the labels revealing the contents of most conditioners, you're looking for a solution to tame your "mane" or your flyaway curls: the richness and creaminess of andiroba oil make it a perfect fit for a simple fix. A few drops of pure oil applied to the full length of your hair make for an efficient, nourishing, detangling conditioner.

ANDIROBA-BASED RECIPES

from Officine Universelle

SOOTHING
ANTI-MOSQUITO BALM

At your own risk, you are about to dine outside in the warmth of a summer evening, in a setting that is as tempting for the mosquitoes as it is for you. . . .

Three tablespoons plus one teaspoon of andiroba oil mixed with three drops each (or ½ teaspoon) of lemongrass and geranium essential oils will efficiently deter insects. This liquid can be prepared in a small jar equipped with a dropper and applied, just before you step outside, on your arms, legs, nape, and neckline area. Wait for your skin to absorb the oil before you put on your dress or your shirt.

DRAINING MASSAGE OIL

Summer beckons, bikini season is around the corner, and you have lowered your sugar intake. Stack the odds in your favor with a daily massage using this draining oil.

In a small jar equipped with a dropper, mix one part andiroba oil with one part tamanu oil, and generously massage this fluid into the more "padded" parts of the body.

Be patient; this treatment requires a bit of persistence: "Rome wasn't built in a day."

⊹ APRICOT ⊹

Powder, natural oil — Origin: Armenia

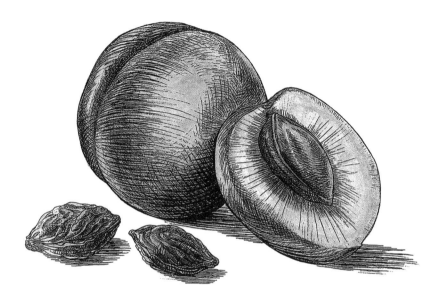

Prunus armeniaca

SOFT DRUPE

○

In springtime, *Prunus armeniaca* — a diminutive, robust tree native to Central and East Asia — adorns itself with small deciduous leaves, followed by pearly white blossoms and tender fruit: apricots. Armenia is the other cradle of the apricot tree, which now comes in thousands of varieties, cultivated for this tiny, oh-so-plump, downy fruit, with its extremely delicate orange color and marvelous aroma. Saying that a cheek has an apricot complexion is a compliment that imparts an even rosier glow to its happy recipient, given the radiant, velvety appearance of this pretty fruit. Between this epidermal analogy and the idea of turning the apricot into a beauty care product lies a long history.

TEACHINGS FROM TIME IMMEMORIAL

○

Traditional Chinese medicine uses apricot as an ingredient in longevity elixirs. Nicknamed "lucky fruit," the apricot's stones, whose very hard shells contrast with the fruit's tenderness, were finely milled using a mortar and pestle and mixed with other medicinal powders. As for the oil, it is obtained by pressing the kernels inside that stone. The most well-known product is probably that of the apricot trees grown on the spectacular terraces of the Kashmiri mountains. The Hunza or Burusho people, horticulturists by trade, are still reputed to live past one hundred and their spirited longevity is attributed to their fruit-and-vegetable-rich diet, in which the apricot, under its many guises, plays a central role.

ON COLLECTING APRICOT KERNEL OIL

◦

Oil is the most ingenious product to be derived from the apricot. The extremely hard and rugged stones within the fruit are opened, and the kernels they contain are crushed to extract a thousand benefits. Forty to 45% of the kernel is made up of an orangey-yellow oil. Luminous and sunny, this finely textured oil gives out a mild scent, reminiscent of the aroma of bitter almond (*Prunus dulcis*). The Mediterranean basin is now the world's largest apricot orchard. Turkey is the number one producer of apricots: the fruit harvested there is, for the most part, destined to be dried and used as food.

THE BENEFITS

◦

Apricot kernel oil is reputed to enhance the cheeks' rosy glow and to tighten the skin's grain. It contains an impressive concentration of fatty acids: between 60 and 70% oleic acid (omega-9) and between 20 and 25% linoleic acid (omega-6). Its vitamin A content is particularly high: it fosters cellular turnover and helps brighten the complexion. Over in the West, Mr. Jean Valnet, a celebrated French phytotherapy expert and a pioneer of plant-based medicine, promotes the use of apricot juice to tone normal skin, because of its rather astringent, regenerative properties.

"One bite of the immortality fruit is better than a whole indigestion of apricots."

CHINESE PROVERB

JUST A FEW DROPS

Do you prefer city lights to the morning sun and walks out in the open? A few drops of apricot kernel oil, massaged directly onto the face, will fend off any allusion to the benefits of sleep to keep you looking fresh. . . . This oil will maintain adequate hydration levels for your skin and will greatly boost your complexion!

APRICOT-BASED RECIPES

from Officine Universelle

APRICOT AND ROSE PURIFYING AND STIMULATING MASK

For those difficult, dull, and sensitive skin mornings — a weekly lifesaver!

Enhanced with a teaspoon of apricot kernel oil and two teaspoons of rose water, two generous tablespoons of red clay will make a mask that has a balancing, purifying, and reviving effect on dull skin and uneven complexions. Apply a thick layer of this mask and leave it on for five to seven minutes. Carefully rinse with warm water and gently pat dry with a soft cloth.

You're glowing!

FACIAL RADIANCE OINTMENT

To be used on a summer Sunday, this concoction will give you a rosy complexion to match your bathing suit. You'll have to pinch a couple of ripe apricots from the kitchen before they end up in a pie. Leave this sweet-and-sour mask on as you lie down to rest in the shade of a tree, or as you sit comfortably in a bathroom with a view.

Crush the flesh of two good-looking apricots and collect their refined pulp in a small bowl. Add one teaspoon of apricot kernel oil and one of rose water. Mix until you obtain a soft paste, to be applied directly to the face and neckline. Leave for ten minutes before rinsing off with fresh water. Pat the skin dry with a clean, dry towel and finish by applying a few drops of apricot kernel oil.

⬥ ARGAN ⬥

Vegetable oil (kernels) — Origin: Morocco

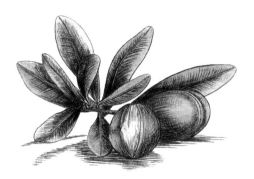

Argania spinosa

THE THOUSAND-
YEAR-OLD TREE

◉

*A*rgania spinosa, a small tree from the Sapotaceae family, yields fruit containing a protective pulp surrounding a nut, which itself shelters a varying number of seeds. Often celebrated as the "tree of life" or the "thousand-year-old tree," the argan tree is a relic from the Tertiary period. It is native to Morocco and, to a lesser extent, Algeria. It is now mostly grown in the Souss Valley in southwestern Morocco, a region that is simultaneously oceanic and arid, where this small but robust tree, with its round top and knotty trunk, has adapted magnificently to the poor soil. Sadly, the treasure that is the great Moroccan argan grove is being depleted by the activity and population increases of both humans and animals.

TEACHINGS FROM TIME
IMMEMORIAL

◉

Argan oil is a panacea of which humans have been aware for thousands of years. The Egyptian physician Ibn al-Baytar mentioned argan in his *Compendium on Simple Medicaments and Foods* (1219) under the name of *ârjânet lûz al-bârabîr* — the Berber almond. It has long been in use by the Berber people from the rare countries in which the argan tree still thrives naturally, sheltered from intensive agriculture. Valued by modern cosmetology, it has become an ingredient in cosmetic products, but it is never as soothing or potent as when it is pure — applied directly to the skin and hair, the way women have been using it since the dawn of time. . . .

LEGENDARY BEAUTY

◉

The power of argan is ancient and renowned. It crossed paths with Tin Hinan — a legendary, stunningly beautiful queen, made famous in a novel by Pierre Benoit in which she is called Antinea. Concealed in her desert palace, on the blue slopes of the Atlas Mountains in southern Morocco, Antinea shields her fabulous beauty. On the starriest nights, dressed in almost nothing, she goes horseback riding into the desert in search of fresh air. During one of these far-flung nighttime excursions, her stallion throws her off and gallops away. The sun rises as Antinea is walking east, her skin soon cruelly touched by its ardent glare. She finds relief in the shade of a few diminutive trees. Their branches bear fruit protected by a rind which, once broken, reveals three kernels. She eats a few of them and uses a stone to crush others on a rock in order to anoint her tired skin with the resulting oil. Once her burns are soothed, she falls asleep. The next day, her skin looks fresh and radiant again, thanks to the miraculous tree. Antinea sets off on her return journey. Once back in her gardens, she plants the seeds of the argan tree and concocts a secret ointment to preserve her beauty: argan oil.

ON COLLECTING ARGAN OIL

The small fruits of the argan tree are pulpy, bright yellow, and spindle shaped. Each contains an especially hard nut that holds two or three kernels. Carefully shelled and peeled by expert, often feminine hands, they are cold-pressed to obtain a pungent, bright yellow oil. Argan oil has a naturally fine texture. For cosmetic use, purchasing oil obtained from pre-roasted kernels is not recommended; this oil is better suited for cooking than beauty treatments. The color of the oil should be pale, and its aroma shouldn't be strong enough to irritate you. This would be a sign that the kernels were either already spoiled when they were harvested, or that they were treated improperly.

THE BENEFITS

Argan oil contains potent natural active ingredients: tocopherols or vitamin E (antioxidants that help protect cells from the oxidation caused by free radicals), sterols that foster microcirculation, and palmitic acid and stearic acid that assist with oxidation. Not only is it exceptionally healthy, it is also wonderfully flavorful. Argan oil is highly regarded and has somewhat of a magical aura in the Souss Valley, where it is given to guests as a welcoming present.

JUST A FEW DROPS

This precious oil is often victim to its popularity as a hair care remedy, which has cast a shadow over its numerous other uses. As a facial treatment, argan oil alleviates wrinkles and the dark spots that come with aging. It can heal dry skin and even superficial injuries. A few drops, applied to burns, will help them scar over.

Because it reduces inflammation, it is also able to gradually soothe the discomfort caused by acne. To this end, argan oil should be applied on freshly cleansed skin with all traces of makeup removed. Its use is also recommended on chickenpox blisters: it is known to help them scar over, and to prevent secondary infections.

ARGAN OIL–BASED RECIPES

from Officine Universelle

ANTIOXIDANT
HEALING FACIAL SERUM

Once a day, or on evenings marked by great fatigue, tend to morale and skin with this deliciously scented elixir.

In a small jar with a dropper filled with three tablespoons plus one teaspoon of argan oil, dispense six drops (or ½ teaspoon) of rose essential oil, or neroli essential oil if you prefer its honeyed aroma. Mix by gently shaking the flask. You now have an exquisitely scented elixir that bestows youth and radiance.

Long live the natural finery of soft, smooth, well-hydrated, and rested skin.

TREATMENT MASK
FOR THE FACE AND CHEST

It is time to get some clarity—in the mind as well as the skin. . . . Rhassoul works wonders to balance and treat uneven, tired complexions.

In a small bowl, mix one tablespoon of argan oil and a fistful of rhassoul clay with three tablespoons of geranium hydrolate. Leave this purifying treatment on for five to ten minutes, rinse copiously without rubbing the skin, and pat dry using a clean towel.

This treatment cleanses deeply: after applying this mask, be sure to hydrate the skin again using one or two drops of argan oil.

ARGAN OIL–ENHANCED
SHAMPOO

Why not improve on a product you purchased: on-the-spot salves are your ticket to custom-made care.

In a small metal bowl, combine one measure of organic shampoo with one "palmful" of water (the amount of water you can hold in one cupped hand) and four to six drops of argan oil, depending on the length and thickness of your hair. Blend the mixture in the bowl and pour it on your head, then gently massage your scalp using your fingertips rather than your nails, even if shampooing has made your scalp itchy. Always rinse carefully, and towel dry without rubbing.

✦ ARNICA ✦

Flowers and rhizomes — Origin: Central Europe

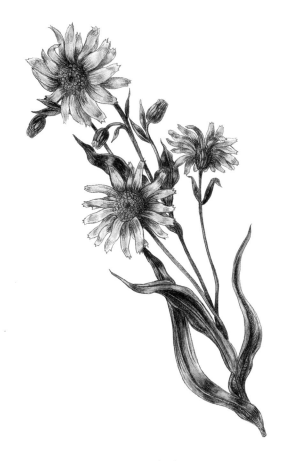

Arnica montana

THE PANACEA OF BUMPS AND BRUISES

◉

*A*rnica montana, the emblematic yellow flower of the mountains of Central Europe, is a perennial plant that thrives in elevated meadows and wild prairies. Its intrepid and hardy rhizomes can withstand the harshness of winter at high altitudes.

TEACHINGS FROM TIME IMMEMORIAL

◉

The use of arnica in phytotherapy has long been documented. The famed Pedanius Dioscorides nicknamed it *alcimos*, i.e., "healthy." In the 14th century, in his *Commentarii* on the works of the aforementioned Greek physician and botanist, Matthioli mentioned it under its

> *"Time soon spread the arnica of oblivion over my wounded heart."*

ALPHONSE ALLAIS

current name, *arnich*. In 1625, arnica was cited in Jakob von Bergzabern's botany treatise for the same properties that we attribute to it today: caring for bruises after minor bumps and falls. Its sylvan and fantastical German name, *Bergwohlverleih* ("wolf killer"), which sounds straight out of a fairy tale, is testament to the danger the plant poses to certain animals. One might wonder what kind of wolf would be willing to bite into it. . . . According to popular belief, arnica was associated with the demonic eyes of that carnivorous beast, which it was reputed to control. The *Kornwolf*, or grain wolf, was said to roam through the cornfields. It symbolized the field's vitality as well as the spirit of the grain. To prevent this wolf from straying off, and the crop from withering away, farmers would plant arnica seedlings along the fields' edges on Saint John's Day, the summer solstice. Arnica was also reputed to protect the harvest from *Bilwisschnitter*, the grain demon. It was even considered a protection against the damage wrought by storms and lightning.

Goats, on the other hand, are reported to graze instinctively on arnica after a fall: this habit is said to have brought the plant's properties to their shepherds' attention. In the Vosges Mountains, it was customary to smoke dried arnica leaves and flowers in lieu of tobacco. In the Alps, its leaves, cooked in wine, used to be applied as poultices. Arnica is one of the plants that are most emblematic of phytotherapy's expansion: it proved highly inspirational to Samuel Hahnemann, the founder of homeopathy, and today it is one of the most commonly used plants in alternative medicine.

ON PREPARING ARNICA

The flower is plucked shortly after blooming, in May and June. After centuries of being harvested in the wild, it was included in the Washington Convention's list of species endangered by man. Therefore, its harvest is now subject to regulation in numerous countries. The flowers macerate for a few weeks in a neutral oil, which then takes on a fine orange tint and a warm, gentle scent.

THE BENEFITS

The flavonoids it contains help fortify blood vessels and stimulate blood circulation. Antiseptic thymol, draining coumarin, soothing carotenoids, and anti-inflammatory sesquiterpene lactones help damaged and irritated skin recover its peace and vitality.

A FEW DROPS

Arnica macerate is an indispensable addition to every family's medicine cabinet. It should be applied with care to gently heal bruises, cramps, and sprains. Massaged onto the skin, it proves extremely useful in recovering from, or better preparing for, sports-related exploits.

ARNICA-BASED RECIPES
from Officine Universelle

RASPBERRY SEED OIL–BASED ARNICA MACERATE

Does your skin get irritated at the slightest provocation? Have you overindulged in the sun? Do you crave rosy cheeks after the paleness of winter? This fluid will work wonders.

Fill a small jar with a wide mouth up to its middle with dried arnica flowers, then cover these with raspberry seed oil. Seal the jar so it is airtight and allow to macerate for four weeks, regularly turning the jar over. Filter through cotton gauze (for instance, an unfolded bandage), while pressing the flowers so as not to waste any of the macerate, then pour the oil into a sterilized, airtight container.

"Set fire to the arnica and the weather will turn."

GERMAN PROVERB

⊹ AVOCADO ⊹

Oil, pulp (pulp) — Origin: Mexico

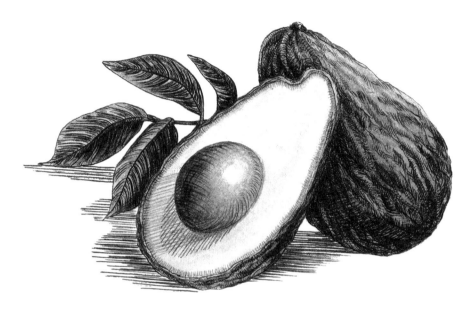

Persea americana

"ALLIGATOR PEAR"

◦

The avocado, with its pale yellow and light green pulp, blossoms on the *Persea americana*, an evergreen whose oldest variety appears to originate from Mexico. At the core of this gentlest of fruits, beloved for its delicate flesh, grows a very large pit, which used to be grated and incorporated into the making of beauty treatments. Nowadays, the most widely grown variety is a cross between the hardy Mexican avocado and its cousin from Guatemala, which grows as far away as New Zealand. Unusually, its fruit is harvested while still green and doesn't ripen until after the harvest.

TEACHINGS FROM TIME IMMEMORIAL

◦

The ubiquity and consumption of this fruit, which was highly prized by the Aztecs and the Maya, have been documented thanks to the excavation of numerous archeological sites, where researchers have exhumed fossilized avocado pits of all sizes. Such abundance and diversity are said to reflect the careful selection and cultivation of bigger, more beautiful fruit. The first Westerner known to have mentioned the avocado was the Spanish geographer Martín Fernández de Enciso in a book published in 1518–19. However, this exotic fruit would not reach Europe until the 17th century. The peoples of Central America nourished themselves with its appetizing pulp, which they believed had aphrodisiac properties, and used it to beautify their hair.

ON COLLECTING AVOCADO OIL

o

The extraction of avocado oil entails a highly delicate and technical process, which aims to separate water from the beneficial oil contained in the fruit's flesh. One way to do this is to dehydrate shavings of avocado by applying moderate heat and then to press them and collect the oil. Another process involves centrifugation of the fruit's pulp, followed by cold-pressing. A good avocado oil should have a deep green tint and exude a fresh and unmistakable botanical scent. The texture is always thick and enveloping, but the oil absorbs remarkably well despite its viscosity.

THE BENEFITS

o

The avocado contains numerous potent fatty acids, as well as nutrients whose properties help prevent oxidation. Low in carbohydrates and rich in good lipids (omega-3), it comes highly recommended as part of a healthy diet. It has calming properties in stressful times. Its oil has a high concentration of palmitic acid, whose emollient and hydrating benefits are felt deep within the skin, and of oleic acid (omega-9), which helps with scarring. Avocado oil also contains precious vitamins: H, which fosters hair growth; K, which helps alleviate dark rings around the eyes; and PP, which protects the skin from the ill effects of light. Finally, phytosterols— soothing and antioxidant rich—minimize the damage caused by ultraviolet light from exposure to the sun. Avocado oil is particularly potent on mature or suntanned skin. Used as an ointment on the hair and scalp prior to shampooing, it makes the hair strong and radiant.

A FEW DROPS

Some feminine exploits require efficient and simple treatments. In order to support the feats performed by a pregnant woman's skin, pure avocado oil can be applied daily to care for their curves and prevent the onset of stretch marks. This unctuous oil will leave the skin supple and sufficiently hydrated.

AVOCADO-BASED RECIPES

from Officine Universelle

AVOCADO OIL–BASED NOURISHING HAIR MASK

In beauty, as in literature, there are classics. Some recipes must be tried as part of a well-rounded aesthetic education— this maintenance mask for the hair is one such panacea.

In a small bowl, using a kitchen whisk, thoroughly mix one tablespoon of avocado oil with one or two egg yolks, depending on the length of your hair. Apply this mixture to the mid-lengths and ends. Leave on for about thirty minutes and rinse off with a gentle shampoo.

AVOCADO PULP–BASED FORTIFYING HAIR MASK

This take on a restorative mask for damaged hair calls for regular weekly use to replenish the hair's natural balance.

In a small bowl, using a fork, mash the flesh of a well-ripened avocado, then add the juice of half a lemon and a teaspoon of tamanu oil. Apply the resulting paste to the hair's lengths and ends. Leave on for about thirty minutes. Then wash the hair with a gentle shampoo, diluted with a small amount of warm water.

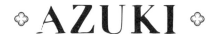

☙ AZUKI ☙

Beans (powder) — Origin: Japan

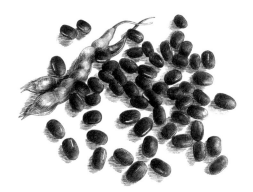

Vigna angularis

THE KING BEAN

○

Vigna angularis is an annual
climbing plant originating from
the Chinese side of the Himalayas.
Its cultivation has been documented across
Asia since before the year 1000. The azuki
(its Japanese name), or red bean, is a tiny
bean that, tightly packed alongside its
brethren, grows in long segmented pods.
In Japan, the most prestigious cultivar
of this "king of beans," the *tamba*, is the
specialty of the Hyogo prefecture. It has a
reputation for a particularly exquisite taste
and a smooth and tender texture. Crushed
to a powder, the beans of *Vigna angularis*
are the main ingredient of a paste that is
widely used in all Asian cuisines, especially
in pastries.

TEACHINGS FROM TIME IMMEMORIAL

○

The delicate, pink-colored powder
obtained from grinding azuki beans has
been used for centuries in Japan and
throughout Asia to cleanse the face gently
and deeply. Fair Japanese ladies used to
rub their faces and bodies with little silk
sachets filled with this powder. Azukitogi,
a well-known *yokai* of Japanese folklore,
is a mischievous spirit who is always
washing azuki beans on the edge of a body
of water: get anywhere near him, and he'll
push you in! In Chinese medicine, azuki
beans are considered a healthy ingredient
whose ingestion is recommended as a
way to get rid of toxins, for instance in
cases of urinary tract infections. It is also
considered a rather fancy food: A Japanese
legend tells the story of a mother who fed
red beans to her son, Fudô-Iwa, and soy
to her stepson, Gongen-Yama. Since the
fancier azuki beans were less nourishing,
her favorite son remained weaker than
his brother. The two enjoyed playing
together. One day, each tied a rope around
his neck, and pulled on the other's rope.
When Gongen pulled, Fudô-Iwa's head
went rolling all the way down to the next
village. . . . The Chinese tradition of eating
azuki porridge to chase away evil spirits
also exists in Korea: *patjuk* is especially
popular on the day of the winter solstice.

ON COLLECTING AZUKI BEANS

This bean matures slowly: it takes about a hundred and twenty days to develop fully. Its harvest occurs in September, when the pods open spontaneously, revealing dark, glossy beans.

THE BENEFITS

The azuki bean is rich in saponins (natural cleansing agents) and in minerals that are beneficial to the epidermis. The proanthocyanidins it has in abundance are potent antioxidants. Its excellent vitamin B concentration helps revive the skin, gives it a certain radiance, and fosters its oxygenation and hydration.

A FEW PINCHES

A pinch of red bean powder, moistened and massaged onto damp oily or combination skin, will gently and efficiently cleanse the face. You can make azuki beans into powder using a mortar and pestle or a coffee grinder.

AZUKI-BASED RECIPES

from Officine Universelle

BALANCING FACIAL MASK

Is your skin going back and forth between scattered blemishes, dilated pores, and dryness? Once a week, take the time to leave this cleansing mask on: it will restore balance.

Mix one tablespoon of red bean powder and one tablespoon of organic honey. Leave on for about twenty minutes. Gently massage your face and rinse.

SOFTEST CLEANSER FOR A STRESSED SCALP

Take advantage of a quiet day to try this gentle cleansing scrub for the scalp, in lieu of your usual corrosive foam.

Massage your scalp with some camellia oil, after dispensing a few drops along a few wide partings. Once the camellia oil has been absorbed, separate the hair into a dozen thick sections, without overlooking the back of your head. Massage a few pinches of azuki powder onto each section. Next, dilute a tablespoon of azuki powder in a large glass of warm water and pour the mixture over all your hair. To complete the massage, emulsify, then rinse at length. Follow by rinsing with some clear water spiked with a little rice vinegar.

☘ BAOBAB ☘

Vegetable oil (seeds) — Origin: Senegal

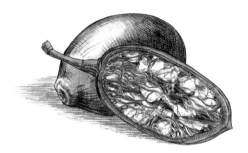

Adansonia digitata

THE UPSIDE-DOWN TREE

Adansonia digitata is the iconic tree of dry, tropical Africa and of the continent's savanna landscapes. It's called the baobab, from the Arabic *bu hibab*, which means "many-seeded fruit"—and these seeds are its most precious riches. Grilled and ground, they are used to brew scrubland "coffee," and when pressed, they yield an oil that possesses highly revered properties. The fruit's pulp, also known as "monkey bread," is very rich in vitamin C and calcium, and can be drunk fresh as a fruit juice. It is known to fortify pregnant women and babies.

TEACHINGS FROM TIME IMMEMORIAL

This tree is sacred; palavers are traditionally held at its foot. People have always been struck by its extraordinary longevity—it is said to live for a thousand years. Its hollow trunk is filled with water. The famed Berber traveler Ibn Battûta was the first to mention the baobab in a 16th-century record of his travels through the Niger River basin. In the day-to-day African pharmacopeia, the baobab is a major resource, and there is a use for all of its parts: its seeds, the pulp of its fruit, its bark, its leaves, and its roots, which are imbued with anti-inflammatory and digestive properties.

ON COLLECTING BAOBAB FRUIT

The fruit of the baobab looks like a large bean. The pulp contains small brown seeds with an orange tint. Cleaned, dried, and crushed, they yield the makings of a paste that has traditionally been prized for softening and nourishing the skin, as well as for healing burns. This paste is carefully strained and then pressed so as to extract a rich oil.

THE BENEFITS

Baobab seed oil is the best friend of dry and exposed skin. Rich in oleic acid (omega-9), it nourishes the skin and fully preserves its elasticity. Its abundance of linoleic acid (omega-6) fosters cell turnover and is even more efficient when combined with the baobab's high concentration of vitamin E, which protects the skin from oxidation. The stearic acid takes care of dry and brittle hair.

JUST A FEW DROPS

The sea air, the wind, and your walks outside do you good. Unfortunately, your skin may not feel the same. . . . In difficult climatic conditions, baobab seed oil soothes skin that is exposed to wind and temperature gradients. Applying a few drops on damp skin in the morning and a few drops on well-cleansed skin at night will intensify the radiance of your complexion. Baobab seed oil protects the skin, nourishes chapped hands, hardens the nails, and prevents or alleviates stretch marks.

BAOBAB SEED OIL–BASED RECIPES

from Officine Universelle

REVIVING MASK
FOR COARSE HAIR

A weekly treatment for very, very dry hair.

Using a fork, mix four teaspoons of baobab seed oil with one teaspoon of castor seed oil, one ounce of soft shea butter and three drops of ylang ylang essential oil, until you obtain an even paste. Apply this concoction to the hair and scalp and leave it on for half an hour, then shampoo twice in a row with hot water and an organic cleanser.

> *"It is easier to uproot a blade of grass from your neighbor's flower pot than a baobab from your own garden."*

BANTU PROVERB

ANTI–STRETCH MARK OIL

The indelible traces of your body's fluctuations are a souvenir you could do without, even if they are reminders of happy occasions. Regular massage will improve the appearance of these unwanted souvenirs and minimize their damage.

In a small jar with a dropper, mix two tablespoons of baobab seed oil, two tablespoons of rose hip seed oil, and six drops of *Helichrysum italicum* essential oil (the latter is also known as "Immortelle," its French nickname). Every day after your morning routine, apply this concoction to the areas that are most affected by pregnancy: your thighs, your stomach, and the backs of your arms.

You're already feeling better: breaking away from certain physical realities can be a morale booster.

✦ BEE ✦

Honey and beeswax — Origin: World

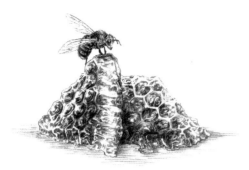

Apis mellifera

"HONEY WITH PLEASURE, A STING WITH REGRET"

◦

Bees make honey from the nectar of flowers or the honeydew. Once the harvest is complete, this material is held in a natural pocket during flight and delivered to the workers, who enrich it and use it to feed the hive.

TEACHINGS FROM TIME IMMEMORIAL

◦

Since prehistory, man has observed the work of the bee and put it to use: apiculture was without a doubt the first type of animal farming to ever be practiced. The hive's organization exerts a certain fascination. The Greek philosopher Aristotle said of bees that "they constitute an exceptional genus." For the ancient Egyptians, honey was a divine and precious food. Under Pharaoh Ramses II, state employees received part of their salary in honey. In an extensive medicinal papyrus that dates back to the same reign and is now kept in Berlin, the author makes numerous references to honey—to heal coughs and cleanse wounds or abscesses. Beeswax is used to make candles, ointments, remedies, soaps, and polish. Hydrophobic and antibacterial, beeswax was also used in mummification, and its commercial value was then higher than that of honey. In the Roman Empire, apiculture was practiced intensively. A Roman writer from the reigns of emperors Claudius and Nero, Lucius Columella, mentions honey in *Le Libri de Re Rustica*, a treatise on rural economy. Volume IX gives practical insights into how to raise bees and benefit from their precious industry. From the mead of the northern peoples to gingerbread, the culinary uses of honey are numerous, in all civilizations and across all eras. Closer to home, a surprising beauty preparation attributed to Madame de Sévigné, inspired by a recipe from the Salerno School, recommends incorporating bee ash into rose oil to care for the hair.

ON COLLECTING HONEY

◦

When the honey is ripe, bees use wax to obstruct the hive cell in which it is stored, the better to safeguard this precious food reserve. To extract the honey from the hive, the apiculturist will either smoke or blow the bees out temporarily. The frames, stacked side by side within the hive, are removed and transferred to a protected, dry place. The cells' protective wax is removed, and the honey flows out of the cells. At the time of harvest, all types of honey are liquid; some of them—depending on the nature of the flowers from which they were made—later congeal more than others. The frames are placed in an extractor, and all the honey is then finely strained to remove any waxy residue. It is recommended to let honey mature for a year to enjoy the full richness of its aroma. It can keep for many years without going bad.

THE BENEFITS

Beeswax is composed of wax esters: monoesters, diesters, triesters, hydroxipolyesters, and hydroximonoesters, which form a protective film on the skin. Rich in vitamin A, wax accelerates cell turnover and can help improve patchy skin. The propolis contained in the wax also has well-known antibacterial properties.

As for honey, it contains a very large quantity of sugars (fructose, glucose, and saccharose),

which capture water molecules and protect the skin from drying out. It is also rich in an enzyme which is able to synthesize hydrogen peroxide, an antibacterial substance. Its high concentration of mineral salts (whose composition varies) and of vitamins B1, B2, B3, B5, B6, and B9 deeply nourish and regenerate the skin. Its amino acids help cleanse the skin and accelerate the process of scarification.

A FEW DROPS

Honey is remarkable and boasts great cosmetic qualities. It is an excellent base for preparations that absorb, preserve, and transmit the properties of plants. In the winter, to heal chapped lips, apply some honey, just barely diluted with a little floral water, as often as required. All honeys are different: acacia honey is soothing; honey made from chestnut flowers stimulates blood circulation; made from heather flowers it is particularly rich in mineral salts; lavender honey is famously antiseptic; that of Manuka is antibacterial and anti-inflammatory; thyme honey helps with scarification; and rosemary honey soothes eczema. One should always choose a honey that derives from organic agriculture.

HONEY-BASED RECIPES
from Officine Universelle

RADIANT BEAUTY
SOFTENING MASK

Easy to use and always available in the kitchen, honey leaves the skin softened and soothed. Its texture can be tamed through the addition of natural oils.

Using a fork, mix a tablespoon of honey, the juice of half a lemon, and a few drops of camellia oil. Apply this balm directly to dry skin, and leave on for fifteen minutes. Gently massage with warm water, and rinse off.

SOS OINTMENT
FOR ACNE

Have your cheeks, forehead, chin, and the sides of your nose fallen victim to a sudden outbreak? This heroic mask can help reduce the inflammation and bring relief.

In a small bowl, using a bamboo whisk, emulsify one tablespoon of lavender honey, two drops of geranium essential oil, one teaspoon of nigella oil, and three pinches of ground cinnamon. Using a cosmetic brush, apply this mask directly to the inflamed areas of the face and leave on for at least ten minutes. Gently rinse with warm water. Pat dry with a clean, dry cloth, without rubbing the skin. Finish this treatment by applying three drops of nigella oil.

STRENGTH AND SHINE
HAIR BALM

A treatment for lackluster hair, whatever the cause – whether stress, capillary error, or cosmetic excess. A few weekly applications will reverse the trend.

Using a bamboo whisk, mix one tablespoon of liquid honey, one tablespoon of hemp oil, two tablespoons of horsetail hydrolate, and two drops of ylang ylang essential oil. This balm should be applied to clean, damp hair. Leave on for half an hour, then carefully rinse with cool to tepid water.

⬩ BORAGE ⬩

Oil (seeds) — Origin: Europe

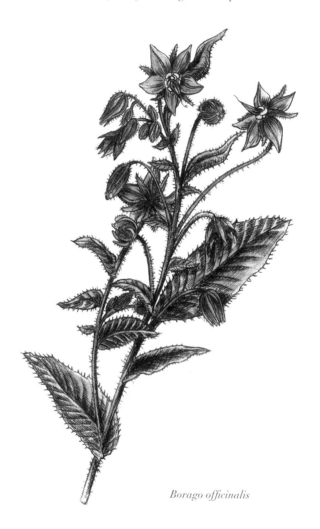

Borago officinalis

A TROVE OF MODESTY

B orage is a very hardy common weed, native to Europe and the whole Mediterranean basin. This "simple" herb, as famous as it is modest, is known by many colorful local aliases:

common bugloss, bee bread, starflower, ox's tongue. . . . Its tall stems, covered in a beautiful fuzz of thick silver hairs, sprout tiny, edible, star-shaped flowers that taste delicious and range from purple and blue to pale pink. Harvested and left to dry, these make for a healthy and detoxifying herbal tea. In recent years they've been featured, freshly picked, on the plates of a new generation of chefs, who use them as a spice with a fresh iodine taste. Borage seeds are pressed for a calming, antiaging oil that also soothes skin suffering from eczema or prone to dermatitis.

TEACHINGS FROM TIME IMMEMORIAL

The Greeks, who used it to season their wine, nicknamed it *euphrosine*, "that which makes one happy." It can counteract some of the morning-after effects of a few too many drinks the night before. Its name comes from the Arabic *abou rach*, "father of sweat," in reference to its sudorific properties, which are held to be purgative and hence beneficial. In the Middle Ages, borage was consumed fresh, and it was believed to have aphrodisiac properties. According to the English herbalist John Gerard in 1597, "Syrup made of the flowers of borage comforts the heart, purges melancholy, and quiets the frenetic and lunatic person." Nowadays, borage oil is often packaged in capsules and recommended for women due to its ability to balance the hormonal system. Borage oil works wonders on the skin from youth through to maturity.

ON COLLECTING BORAGE OIL

So as to ensure the oil's quality, borage seeds are harvested when they reach maturity and take on a brown (rather than green) tint. This oil is cold-pressed, then decanted and carefully filtered. It should exude a pungent aroma but never a rancid one. It is recommended to buy this oil in small quantities and to use it quickly.

THE BENEFITS

Borage oil is rich in linoleic acid (omega-6), which protects the skin from outside stress and efficiently prevents it from drying out. Its high concentration of oleic acid (omega-9) nourishes and helps heal small injuries as well as alleviates itchiness.

A FEW DROPS

Benevolent borage oil brings solace to female skin in particular. It takes care of sensitive, irritated, and reactive skin types; it alleviates psoriasis and atopic dermatitis, and helps smooth over little wrinkles.

"Take the borage but don't tear it off: its flower will heal your heartache and loss."

FRENCH PROVERB

BORAGE-BASED RECIPES
from Officine Universelle

MIRACLE SOOTHING FLUID FOR THE FACE AND NECKLINE
Wrinkles, no matter how small, are sometimes unwanted realities that come with the joy of growing up. . . . A few drops of this fluid will take care of skin that has become mature and sensitive.

In a very small jar with a dropper, mix one part borage oil with one part calendula macerate, enhanced (just for the fun of it) with three drops of ylang ylang essential oil. This should be applied at night, after you've removed every last trace of makeup, by gently rubbing the face and neck.

BORAGE FLOWER BEAUTY BATH
It's important to do things on a grand scale, such as spend a weekend in the countryside looking for fountains and flowers. A simplified version of this youth elixir can be made using our small cotton bag and your bathwater.

In a treatise entitled *Toilette de flore, à l'usage des dames* ("Bathing with flowers, for women's use"), written in 1771, eminent botanist Pierre Joseph Buchoz recommended a borage flower–based beauty bath to soften the skin in what he called "fountain water."

In an extremely hot bath, drop five fistfuls of borage flowers, two fistfuls of hulled barley, and two more of pulverized lupin flowers and bran. . . . Let these ingredients infuse the water as you wait for the bath to cool down. Once it has reached a pleasant temperature, step in — obviously, you should already be clean; taking a shower beforehand will do the trick — and relax for about twenty minutes, to emerge younger and happier!

DRY, FAIR HAIR ENHANCER
A new take on the Sunday hair treatment.

Using a small bamboo whisk, thoroughly mix one tablespoon of borage oil with an egg yolk and one tablespoon of linden hydrolate. For a flawless salve, whisk the yolk before slowly adding the oil and hydrolate. Apply from the scalp to the tips of the hair. Leave on for half an hour, then gently wash your hair.

⟡ BRAZIL NUT ⟡

Oil (nut) — Origin: Amazonia

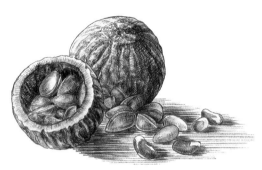

Bertholletia excelsa

LORD OF THE SLOW-PACED

○

With a height of 164 feet, this centenarian tree, *castanheiro do Parà*, dominates the Amazon rain forest from Peru to Ecuador. Its growth is so slow that it's rarely cultivated—it's a real test of patience. All the same, Amerindian cultures have always protected it. Its fruit, known as *pixidios*, or "hedgehogs," is impressive: weighing up to 4.4 pounds, it falls from its branches with a great crash—and more than a little danger! At the core, protected in separate sections, are about ten little nuts. The agouti, a small and greedy rodent who is adept at prying them open, sometimes drops a few along the way, allowing the tree to spread its seeds. Orchid bees are the only insects capable of pollinating them. Harvesting the Brazil nut is an important source of revenue for the populations of Amazonia, who thereby help to preserve the forest— the only possible habitat for this tree.

TEACHINGS FROM TIME IMMEMORIAL

○

The nut of *Bertholletia excelsa*, of which Bolivia is the number one producer, has always been a favored ingredient for the locals and is still sometimes used as currency. Its high oil content also makes it a natural candle. Its shell makes an herbal tea that is said to treat stomach aches. Juan Álvarez Maldonado, a Spanish conquistador and governor of New Andalusia in Peru, fed his troops with this highly calorific nut. Its commodification goes back a long way. Dutch merchants and seafarers were already exporting it to Europe in the 18th century.

In the Tefés tribe, there was once a singularly beautiful and brave maiden. This fair warrior, who went by the name of Caboré, brought luck and prosperity to her people. One day, she went hunting and failed to come back by nightfall. The next morning, the whole tribe set out looking for her, but she was nowhere to be found. Apia, the shaman's son, who was in love with Caboré, refused to stop looking. Exhausted, the warrior sat down on the bank of a river and started crying, imploring the god Tupã to reveal to him the whereabouts of his beloved. Suddenly, he got a glimpse of Caboré's inanimate body reflected in the river and heard a voice explain: "She entered Jurupari territory and was vanquished by evil spirits, but she has become a beautiful and resilient tree," sowing her seeds of luck throughout the forest and feeding her people for all eternity: *La Castanheira*.

in the sun, or in a low-temperature oven. They are so rich that they require just one pressing to yield an abundant, very pale yellow oil with a sweet, nutty scent, which solidifies in temperatures below 50°F.

ON COLLECTING BRAZIL NUT OIL

◦

Harvesting this highly prized nut remains a rudimentary process, even though it is a very popular export. The hulls are nevertheless simply picked up from the ground at the start of the rainy season. Extraordinarily fragile, very prone to rot and insect attacks, the nuts are thrown into the water as a precautionary measure in order to check their density and quality. If they float instead of sinking, they are unfit for eating and are discarded. The good nuts are then opened and left to dry

THE BENEFITS

◦

The Brazil nut is simultaneously prized and feared because of its high concentration of selenium, a trace element that has antioxidant properties—much like the squalenes it also contains. It holds copious amounts of vitamin E, which protects cells from free radicals, and of vitamin F, which prevents drying and helps fortify the hair. Stearic acid and palmic acid—a major component of the cutaneous barrier—hydrate the skin, while phytosterols minimize inflammation.

"The nut belongs to whoever picks it up."

PORTUGUESE PROVERB

A FEW DROPS

Especially beneficial for long brown hair, whether it is coarse or curly, two or three drops of Brazil nut oil warmed up between your palms can be applied along the full length of the hair and to the tips. This morning maintenance ritual can become a habit, much like the application of your moisturizer.

BRAZIL NUT–BASED RECIPES

from Officine Universelle

FORTIFYING OIL BATH
FOR THE HAIR

A miraculous remedy for deeply unhappy hair, to be used as a seasonal cure.

In a small bowl, using a bamboo whisk, mix vigorously (so as to avoid oxidation) and thoroughly two tablespoons of Brazil nut oil with one egg yolk, two tablespoons of sapote oil, and a few drops of rosemary essential oil. Apply with a brush to the scalp and along the length of the hair and leave on for fifteen minutes as you laze around in your bath; then wash off with a very gentle shampoo.

SPECTACULAR ELBOW,
HAND, AND FOOT SCRUB

A treatment against chronic skin dryness . . .

Using an electric coffee grinder, crush five to seven nuts to a powder; then, in a small bowl, mix with two tablespoons of coconut oil. Vigorously rub this granular fluid on the affected areas. Rinse your feet before you shower to avoid slipping, then step in and rinse off the rest.

Soft as a feather, clean as a whistle.

⬩ BURITI ⬩

Oil (nut) — Origin: South America

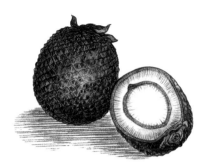

Mauritia flexuosa

A PALM
WITH A THOUSAND USES

○

Mauritia flexuosa is a tall palm tree—and therefore a type of giant grass!—native to the rain forest and found along the banks of the Amazon in marshlands known as *buritizais* or *veredas*. Over the course of several months per year, female palm trees yield a large quantity of fruit. Clustered at the top of the stem—a false trunk—they are protected by a shell that looks like a wonderful dragon egg in the jungle!

TEACHINGS FROM TIME
IMMEMORIAL

○

In the Cerrado, a region of central Brazil, the *buriti*, or "tree of life" to the locals, is sacred. Humans enjoy the fruit as much as macaws, iguanas, and fish, who feed off it happily. Pollination is performed by local bees and small flies.

Its leaves and strong fibers are braided and used to make roofs, baskets, or hats. Young leaves are so supple and thin that they are nicknamed "buriti silk." Musical instruments are carved from the wood of its stem. In the Apinayé tribe, men who are about to be married must prove their strength and skill by carving a chest out of a section of the stem. In the Amazon rain forest, the ripening of the fruit is a cause for celebration, and is also considered to be an auspicious time for weddings. The fruit's bright orange pulp, high in vitamin C, is pressed to extract the juice. The pulp can be cooked into compote or jams. Once fermented, the sap yields a popular type of alcohol, the *vinho de buriti*.

THE STAR TREE

○

History informs us that the Cerrado was peopled by several indigenous tribes. Among them, the most respected was ruled by the Airuana Cacique, and its village belonged to the Tapuia nation on the fertile banks of the Muriti river—the Tapuia name for the Amazon. On starry nights, everyone would gather around the fire to tell stories. During one of these enchanted nights, the chief's youngest daughter, Araci, asked about the birth of the first palm trees that ensured the tribe's prosperity. The old chief explained that after witnessing the harmony of the village, the Creator of all things, Tupa, decided to give the villagers a seed. He named it Muriti and foretold its benefits. To the Krahô Indians, the *buritizeiro* is also a sacred tree, a gift from the fertilizing star Caxekwyj.

ON COLLECTING BURITI OIL

Ripe fruit that has fallen to the ground or bunches that have been cut with a machete are left to dry for several days under the shade of the leaves. Fruit is torn from the bunches and boiled. The intense heat helps separate the pulp from the pit. The pits are then cold-pressed to produce an amazing bright red oil with a sweet and pleasant aroma.

THE BENEFITS

Buriti oil has a high concentration of oleic acid (omega-9). This fatty acid helps with hydration and scarring, and helps restore or preserve the suppleness of the skin. Carotenoids (or pro-vitamin A) minimize the harmful effects of exposure to the sun's rays and calm irritated skin. Vitamin E protects cells from oxidation. Traditionally, the indigenous peoples of the Amazon rain forest would apply this oil to the skin to soothe burns.

"Just because you cannot see the sun does not mean it no longer exists."

AFRICAN PROVERB

A FEW DROPS

Opt for rosy cheeks to fight the gray of early morning and add a drop of buriti oil to your usual facial moisturizer—you'll have chosen an organic option, of course. In the palm of your hand, simply blend a drop of oil with a small teaspoon of cream or liquid and apply delicately. Be aware that buriti oil is a powerful coloring agent—you should always take precautions when using it pure. It can also be diluted in a more neutral oil, such as coconut or jojoba.

BURITI-BASED RECIPES

from Officine Universelle

SEEING RED

Bring some color to your homemade beauty products: in several countries, red symbolizes dynamism and health. It awakens the senses and stimulates blood flow. Kiss your torpor good-bye and say hello to a scarlet body thanks to this exfoliant.

Thoroughly and vigorously mix five tablespoons of buriti oil with six tablespoons of unrefined brown sugar. Migrate to your shower and, sitting on a stool or balanced on one foot, rub the mixture on your skin, taking only a small amount in your hand at a time.

Start with the precious soles of your feet, and work your way up to the base of the neck. Focus on what you are doing and follow your instincts, focusing on the areas that require more than one pass.

And voilà: Your skin is now soft as a feather and temporarily orange-hued, while your well-being positively radiates.

BEAUTIFYING BODY TREATMENT FOR SUN-KISSED SKIN

Enjoy the benefits of buriti oil on your suntanned body by combining it with delicious coconut oil.

In a small jar with a dropper, mix two teaspoons of buriti oil and seven tablespoons of coconut or jojoba oil with eight to ten drops of Atlas cedar essential oil.

One of the great pleasures of summer — sun-kissed, radiant skin.

RADIANCE-RESTORING SHAMPOO FOR DULL, LIFELESS HAIR

For naturally dark, chestnut brown, or red hair, here's a cleansing treatment to apply as often as necessary.

Into a bowl, pour a small quantity of neutral and gentle organic shampoo. Add three drops of buriti oil and mix with a palmful of tepid water. Apply evenly on the hair, wash gently, then rinse.

POST-SUN EMERGENCY TREATMENT

Are you regretting that extra hour at the beach? Time to fix the damage.

In a pharmaceutical vial, mix two teaspoons of buriti oil, ¼ cup of St. John's wort oil, and three drops of true lavender essential oil.

Be sure to love the sun in moderation.

❖ CAMELLIA ❖

Oil (seeds) — Origin: Japan

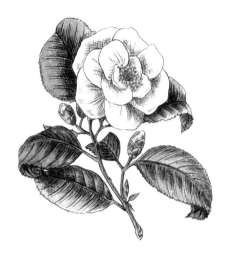

Camellia japonica

THE JAPANESE ROSE
◦

Native to the Himalayas, but thriving as far as Indonesia and Japan, the camellia is an undergrowth shrub whose best-known species is *Camellia sinensis*, the tea tree. The *japonica* variety was acclimatized in Europe in the 17th century. Empress Joséphine de Beauharnais, who had a passion for gardens, made its flowers fashionable and had it planted in the park of the Palace of Malmaison, which harbored hundreds of species and types of new or rare flowers. *Cháhua* in Chinese, *tsubaki* in Japanese, *dongbaek-kkot* in Korean—the camellia's beauty is celebrated globally. Most varieties are ornamental, and their flowers come in a wide array of colors and shapes. Their foliage is dark and glossy. The small flowers of *Camellia japonica* bear capsules that each hold two or three seeds which, when pressed, yield a fine, marvelous oil.

TEACHINGS FROM TIME IMMEMORIAL
◦

The first known mention of camellia oil dates back to 777, when Japan offered some to the ambassador of the Kingdom of Balhae. In *The Tale of Genji*, a Japanese novel from the 11th century, the women of the court use camellia oil to preserve the youthfulness and radiance of their faces and their long black hair. In the Ryoan-Ji Buddhist temple, in Kyoto, you can marvel at a camellia that is said to date back to the 14th century. The tree's branches were used to chase away evil spirits. The arrangement of the flower and its petals, interlocked like those of a compass rose and starched like a piece of fabric, were quick to woo the famous Gabrielle Chanel. The "Great Demoiselle" would soon turn the flower into the triumphant emblem of her modern version of chic.

ON COLLECTING CAMELLIA OIL
◦

Harvesting occurs in September. The fruit is hand-picked from the tree before being steamed; it is then pressed to extract the oil, according to the so-called *tamejime* method. Today, the bulk of (and the finest)

Japanese camellia oil is produced on the Izu Peninsula, about sixty miles from Tokyo. Toshima, where springtime is said to last forever, is famed for the extremely high quality of its tsubaki oil.

THE BENEFITS

Camellia oil has a high concentration of oleic acid, an omega-9 fatty acid that helps preserve the suppleness of the skin. It also accelerates the healing process and soothes damaged skin. Linoleic acid (omega-6), palmitic acid, and stearic acid protect and beautify the hair by coating the hair shafts.

A FEW DROPS

"A woman's hair is her life," a Japanese proverb asserts. Camellia oil is one of the most effective traditional products when it comes to hair care. To sport smooth and shiny hair, with a deep and shimmering color, detangle it calmly and at length using a *tsuge gushi*, a comb made from hard wood, bathed in camellia oil throughout its patient manufacturing process, and later regularly coated with this oil to maintain its beauty and efficacy.

CAMELLIA-BASED RECIPES
from Officine Universelle

NOURISHING AND STRAIGHTENING HAIR-RINSING LOTION

Rinsing is an important and often overlooked step in the process of washing hair. Patient rinsing with fresh water can be enhanced by weekly use of this luster-boosting elixir.

Add two or three drops of camellia oil to a bowl of tepid spring water, along with a dash of lemon juice. Once your hair is washed, whisk the mixture into a salve and rinse your hair with the resulting solution. Pat your hair dry with a clean, dry cloth, without rubbing.

GENTLEST FACIAL CLEANSING MASK

An efficient treatment for the days when you long for a clear, smooth complexion.

Using a small bamboo whisk, carefully mix one teaspoon of camellia oil with one tablespoon of honey and three drops of lemon juice. Leave on your face for a few minutes, then gently massage before rinsing with tepid water. Pat your face dry with a clean, dry cloth.

CASTOR SEED

Oil (seeds) — Origin: Tropical Africa

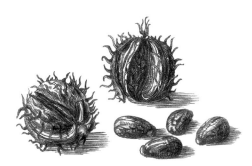

Ricinus communis

CHRIST'S PALM

This tropical shrub is distinguished by its palmate, glossy, and highly decorative leaves, likened to Jesus's hand through the name *Palma Christi*, and which, in India, are associated with elephant ears. The pretty clusters of red and thorny fruits of the castor seed are toxic—they contain a poison which can be lethal if ingested.

TEACHINGS FROM TIME IMMEMORIAL

Castor seed oil has been in use for a very long time—for lighting, making soap, and cleansing the body—thanks to its potent laxative effect. Ayurveda recommends it—under the Sanskrit name of *arandi kaa tel*—mixed with curcuma, for the confection of poultices meant to activate lymphatic circulation. Castor seed oil is one of the world's most widely produced vegetable oils, due to its various cosmetic and pharmaceutical uses. It is unique in that it never congeals, nor freezes.

ON COLLECTING CASTOR SEEDS

The capsule holding the seeds is oval-shaped and protected by a fragile envelope. The seeds' oil content varies depending on the climate: heat increases their size. The fruit ripens under close supervision to prevent the capsules from splitting. Maturation continues while they are left to dry, away from direct sunlight, in order to encourage the capsules to open up. The seeds are separated by simple winnowing or sifting, and are then cold-pressed—unfortunately, industrial production methods use solvents. Castor seed oil is clear, except in the West Indies—the seeds are boiled in water there, which gives the oil a very dark tint and a new name: black castor oil.

THE BENEFITS

Castor seed oil is made up almost exclusively of ricinoleic acid, which accounts for its impressive viscosity. This fatty acid has the rare power of reducing inflammation, and therefore helps heal many a skin problem. It also fills in the scales that line the hair shafts. Vitamin E, which this oil contains in abundance, helps cells fight oxidative stress and helps maintain healthy hair.

A FEW DROPS

As the *Journal des Demoiselles* recommended in 1910: "Take good care of your hands. Let them be white, and let their epidermis be smooth." If you sleep alone and would like to smooth out patchy skin or chicken pox scars, apply a layer of castor seed oil, don cotton gloves, and let ricinoleic acid go to work through the night. To activate eyelash growth, you may also coat their base with some castor seed oil. Apply it, meticulously but not overzealously, using a cotton swab or a small mascara brush. The next morning, after washing, apply two cotton pads soaked with warm water or cornflower hydrolate to the eyes, which will decongest them and remove any excess oil.

CASTOR SEED–BASED RECIPES

from Officine Universelle

EYEBROW GROWTH SERUM

Are you longing for dramatically seductive eyes, and for eyebrows thick enough to highlight them? Perform this treatment as a seasonal cure.

Using a bamboo whisk, mix one teaspoon of castor seed oil with one teaspoon of Belize rum and massage the eyebrows at length with this preparation, without getting too close to the eyes.

> *"Eyes that are short on eyelashes are just sitting there like imbeciles."*
>
> FULANI PROVERB

"KISS ME" BALM

Winter, love, wind . . . all of these give sensitive lips a hard time. Take good care of them with this miracle balm.

In a ceramic bowl placed in a bain-marie, melt 2½ teaspoons of castor seed oil, 2½ teaspoons of jojoba oil, 2½ teaspoons of shea butter, and 2½ teaspoons of beeswax. Once the mixture has cooled down, and before it congeals, add one drop of peppermint essential oil. Pour into a small sterilized bottle or jar with a screw-on cap. This will keep for a few months in the fridge. Each morning, before leaving home, massage some of this balm onto your lips and around your mouth.

❖ CENTELLA ❖

Flowers and stems, macerate — Origin: India

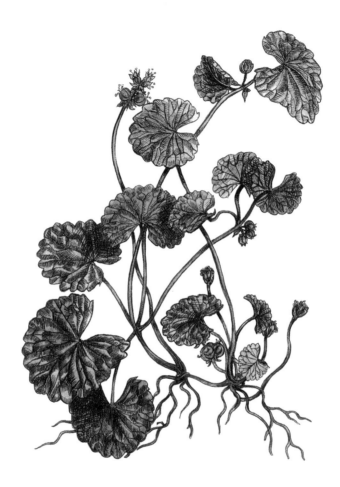

Centella asiatica

"THE TIGER HERB"

Centella asiatica is a perennial semi-aquatic plant bearing beautiful little purple flowers that thrives in the swampy areas of tropical and subtropical countries. Its European variety has none of the medicinal and cosmetic properties of its potent Asian cousin. It has been observed that felines instinctively rub themselves against its foliage when they are wounded. . . .

TEACHINGS FROM TIME IMMEMORIAL

◦

Recognized by all peoples, from India to China, from the Indian Ocean to Melanesia, its potency is harnessed in extracts, ointments, creams, and unguents, in infusions, dressings, and poultices, in mother tinctures and in essential oil. In the *Charaka Samhita*, a famed Sanskrit-language Indian treatise describing three hundred and fifty medicinal plants, the virtues of *Centella asiatica*, or brahmi, are expounded at length. Elsewhere, it is also nicknamed "bowl of water," or *gotu kola*. It is reputed to heal wounds and severe skin conditions; in Madagascar, it is applied to cure the signs of leprosy as well as venous issues. Yogis use it to improve the length and intensity of meditation. In Sri Lanka, *Centella asiatica* is one of the staples of the elephants' frugal and highly selective diet. It has thus acquired the reputation of being a longevity plant. Consuming two of its leaves a day reportedly ensures smooth and healthy aging! It is said that the famous Chinese herbalist Li Ching-Yuen, who is said to have lived past two hundred fifty (!) and had more than twenty spouses, owed his extraordinary longevity to his daily consumption of the plant in infusions and salads, alongside his meditative practice and his frugality. Centella is now a "miraculous" component of so-called smart drinks, as well as an ingredient of numerous hair revitalizers.

ON COLLECTING CENTELLA

◦

The plant's aerial parts are harvested year-round after its first growth spurt in the spring. They are used fresh or dried, and then left to infuse in sesame oil to produce a fine macerate.

THE BENEFITS

◦

Centella asiatica is an ally for those who want to age beautifully; for damaged, exhausted skin; and for lifeless hair. Imbued with antiradical and antioxidant properties, it combines carotenoids, vitamin C, and flavonoids, which stimulate cells, keep them from degenerating, and foster microcirculation within the skin. Saponin, saponosides, polyine, and beta-sistosterol have anti-inflammatory, decongesting, and healing properties.

A FEW DROPS

Centella asiatica macerate is *the* miracle treatment for coarse hair in distress. Used in small amounts, it should be massaged onto the scalp with the tips of your fingers, to stimulate, soothe, and balance. Thanks to transcutaneous absorption, its positive effect on concentration and memory can be expected to complement its benefits for the hair. You may also apply it directly along the length of the hair, and leave this beneficial film on for half an hour or overnight, prior to shampooing. Before going to bed, massage the soles of your feet with this macerate to ensure full relaxation.

CENTELLA-BASED RECIPES

from Officine Universelle

STIMULATING
ANTI–HAIR LOSS SHAMPOO
FOR TIRED HAIR

Our hair ages too: it gets thinner, more brittle, drier, and more fragile. A Centella asiatica cure will allow it to recover some of its luster.

In a small bowl, using a bamboo whisk, blend together ten drops of *Centella asiatica* macerate with one measure of your usual shampoo. Mix with some water and proceed to shampoo your hair. Adopt this treatment for ten to fifteen days.

SOOTHING BALM
FOR DAMAGED AND
IRRITATED SKIN

Take care of yourself as a tiger would and heal minor wounds with Centella asiatica, *in the form of balms and poultices.*

For skin that has been damaged, especially by psoriasis outbreaks, mix ½ ounce of

Centella asiatica leaf powder with seven tablespoons of rose hip seed oil in a small jar. Allow to macerate in a cool (but not cold) place for at least one day, then massage directly onto the skin.

ECZEMA EMERGENCY
POULTICE

Is your skin acting up to get your attention? Breathe deeply to recover a measure of healing calm, then treat the painful area without further delay.

To soothe and heal areas afflicted by eczema, prepare a poultice using two large teaspoons of *Centella asiatica* powder mixed with five teaspoons of mineral water. Leave on for fifteen minutes, protecting the preparation with a soft cloth, and relax as you wait for it to do its job.

"Keep a tranquil heart, sit like a turtle,
walk briskly like a pigeon, and sleep like a dog."

LI CHING-YUEN

❖ CHAMOMILE ❖

Flowers, hydrolate, and essential oil (flowers) — Origin: Central Europe

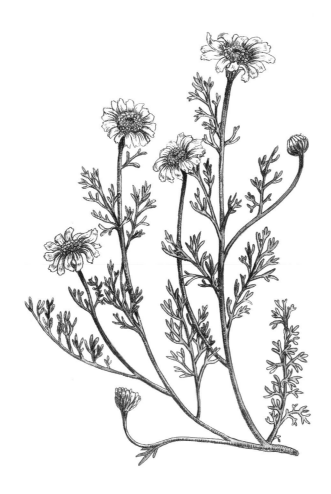

Chamaemelum nobile, Matricaria chamomilla

WILD BEAUTY

❦

This wild herb, whose downy stems are topped by fragrant capitula surrounding a tiny yellow disk, has properties that have been celebrated since antiquity. The Greek name signifies "earth" and "apple," as a nod to its proximity to the former and to the fruity scent of its flowers. Roman chamomile, *Chamaemelum nobile*, and its cousin, *Matricaria chamomilla*, look very similar. The former is often cultivated, the latter more commonly found in the wild.

TEACHINGS FROM TIME IMMEMORIAL

❂

As a symbol of the sun and Ra, the sun god, chamomile was used by the Egyptians in embalming rites as well as in bringing down fevers. In Scandinavian, Saxon, and Nordic mythologies, chamomile numbers among the nine sacred plants that the god Odin supposedly gave mankind. Cultivated by monks in their gardens of "simple" herbs for its therapeutic benefits, it was singled out by Hildegarde de Bingen— the famed 12th-century visionary abbess, magician, and phytotherapist—for its calming effect on digestion and menstrual cramps: "Drink chamomile tea and you will avoid a bellyache." Protective and purifying, chamomile keeps curses at bay when planted around the outside of the house. Some also say that washing one's hands in a chamomile infusion brings good luck to card players.

ON COLLECTING CHAMOMILE FLOWERS

❂

Chamomile flowers are harvested in the summer immediately after blooming. The harvest and the ensuing selection are time-consuming and labor-intensive: four hundred forty pounds of flowers must be plucked to make just eighty-eight pounds of patiently dried flowers! As for the fresh flowers, they are steam-distilled right after the harvest to produce floral water or essential oil. Last but not least, chamomile is also the most widely consumed herbal tea in the world, drunk to calm the spirits and get ready for sleep.

THE BENEFITS

❂

Roman chamomile contains several potent anti-inflammatory active agents: azulene, chamazulene, and flavonoid. Alpha-bisabolol soothes and helps injuries scar over. *Matricaria chamomilla*'s sesquiterpene lactones also soothe inflammation, as do its flavonoids and terpenoids. Chamomile's brightening and softening action on the hair comes from its supply of fructans and terpenoids. It contains azulenes that fight irritation and redness.

A FEW DROPS

There is so much more to do with herbal tea than merely drink it.

An infusion of *Matricaria chamomilla* (two tablespoons in one cup of water) works wonders as a rinse for blond hair, reviving its color and taking care of its health. Do not hesitate to recycle last night's herbal tea in the morning by preparing bags of cold *Matricaria chamomilla* infusion, or soaked compresses. These will soften the area around tired eyes, reduce bags, and un-crumple fragile eyelids.

CHAMOMILE-BASED RECIPES

from Officine Universelle

TEMPER-SOOTHING BATH

There are days when the whole world seems to be ganging up on you. . . . Keep your cool, go home, and draw yourself a bath that will shoo dark thoughts away. And if no bathtub is readily available, don't let it bring you down: welcome a new mood from the outside in by absorbing this remedy through a footbath.

Steep four tablespoons of *Matricaria chamomilla* in two quarts of simmering water; filter this infusion and pour it into a warm bath. Step in, and stay submerged for fifteen minutes.

A romantic comedy? A collection of haikus? You decide on the pastime that will allow you to clear your head and see the world in all its glory.

SOOTHING TREATMENT FOR TEETHING INFANTS

You would do anything to spare your child from this inevitable ache. This combination of floral waters will help.

In a small spray bottle, mix three tablespoons plus one teaspoon of Roman chamomile hydrolate and three tablespoons plus one teaspoon of lavender floral water. One or two pumps sprayed straight into the child's mouth will relieve the inflammation in the gums.

You may also want to try a marshmallow chew stick: giving these new teeth something to work on will bring them comfort.

CLARIFYING, FORTIFYING NAIL BATH

The French version of "A leopard is known by his spots" is "À l'ongle on connaît le lion": "A lion is known by its nails." Do not take yours for granted: this weekly treatment (which beauty dilettantes may resort to monthly) will make them stronger and prettier.

Bathe both hands in seven tablespoons of chamomile hydrolate, enhanced with the juice of a freshly squeezed lemon. After this bath, massage your nails and cuticles with some castor seed oil.

"Liaisons start with champagne and end with chamomile."

VALERY LARBAUD

☙ CHAULMOOGRA ☙

Oil — Origin: India and Myanmar

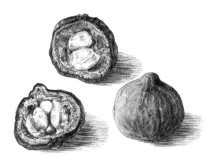

Taraktogenos kurzii

THE MIRACLE TREE

Chaulmoogra is the common name for an Asian family of trees. Among those, *Taraktogenos kurzii* produces the most renowned oil. Himalayan monkeys and black bears are partial to its round, sweet-pulped fruit, which they devour in great quantities. In the past, harvesting took place within the forest as soon as the fruit had fully matured, which took some courage, since this corresponded to the tigers' rutting period — a risky activity, but absolutely worth it.

TEACHINGS FROM TIME IMMEMORIAL

For centuries, as documented in Ayurvedic texts and in the Chinese pharmacopeia, chaulmoogra oil was reputed to cure leprosy. Although it does improve the patient's condition, it cannot singlehandedly halt the disease. An Indian tale, relayed by the

Buddha, says that Rama, King of Benares, had contracted leprosy. As his physicians were unable to cure him, the forlorn king retreated deep within a forest, and found refuge inside a millenary tree, in which he planned to await his end. He fed on the fruit, leaves, and roots of this *kalaw* — the Indian name for the chaulmoogra. Days passed, and it started to seem as if this diet was curing him of his ailment. One night, the king heard the heartrending cries of a girl who was being chased by a tiger: she turned out to be a leper, the daughter of King Oksagarit, and she had found shelter in a cave. Rama killed the beast, brought the girl to his refuge, and had her eat the fruit of the healing tree. The legend adds, in a happy epilogue, that she went on to bear him thirty-two sons. . . . Rama the wise, now cured, elected to stay in the forest where he had recovered his health, and to found a new city.

With his *Hortus Malabaricus,* Hendrik van Rheede, governor of the coastal region of Malabar, penned the first botanical encyclopedia of Southern India. This precious document mentions the benefits of chaulmoogra oil in treating pruritus and other epidermal ailments. In the 19th century, Frederic John Mouat, an English physician, performed the first clinical trials at a Calcutta hospital. Father Raimbault, a botanist priest from the first half of that century, cured his patients with (highly painful) injections of chaulmoogra oil.

ON COLLECTING THE OIL

Overall production fluctuates widely: a bountiful harvest one year is often followed by several years of meager fructification. The oil is extracted by pressing the ripe, fresh kernels after washing, drying, and crushing. Its texture is dense and half-solid, and its aroma very pungent.

THE BENEFITS

Chaulmoogra contains a rare antibacterial and antimycobacterial blend of hydnocarpic and gorlic acids, as well as chaulmoogric acid, which has the same properties and can help regulate the skin's pigmentation. Oleic acid (or omega-9) and palmitic fatty acid help the skin stay hydrated and supple.

A FEW DROPS

This potent oil is a perfect treatment to even out the complexion after a summer of sunbathing, and to ward off the apparition of sunspots. Nowadays, its use against cellulite is generating renewed interest in this little-known oil: pour about ten drops of chaulmoogra oil in the palm of your hand and liquefy them with a few drops of jojoba oil. Massage this blend deeply into the body's padded areas. Perform this massage every day as a month-long cure.

CHAULMOOGRA-BASED RECIPES

from Officine Universelle

ANTI-ITCH BALM

In periods of stress, this will fight bouts of eczema and psoriasis.

Prepare a small jar—properly sterilized and thoroughly dry. In a bowl, carefully mix one tablespoon of chaulmoogra oil with two tablespoons of shea butter, three pinches of burdock powder, and ten drops of Roman chamomile essential oil with a fork, until the mixture becomes smooth and even. Fill the little jar and keep it in a cool place. Apply the balm to the affected areas as often as required.

❖ CLAYS ❖

Powder — Origin: World

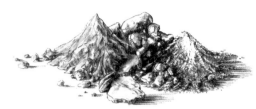

Argilla

THE FIRST MAN

○

Clay is a rock or soil material made up of aluminum and iron silicates, magnesium, calcium, copper, sodium, potassium, manganese . . . and crystallized into very fine particles. After stone and wood, clay, which is present all over the planet in different compositions and hues (white, yellow, pink, red, green, blue, purple . . .), is one of the primordial materials used by men since the dawn of time to build shelters, to craft utensils and garments, and to heal. Its Latin name, *Argilla*, is derived from the Greek *argillos*, meaning "sparkling whiteness"—a nod to the most highly prized of clays, kaolin. The earliest historically documented exploitation of a deposit occurred at a specific Chinese kaolin (*gaoling*, or "soil of the high hills") mine, some two thousand years ago. Clay has been in use since man first became man. So other deposits could claim this honor—if only they could back it up with some documentation. As is often the case, our first uses of this material were inspired by our observations of animal behavior: seeing various beasts roll around with delight and relief in refreshing, healing, and protective clay mud, our ancestors chose this fine material to protect themselves from parasites and the sun, to bandage their wounds, to camouflage themselves and hunt unseen, to wash themselves, and so on.

TEACHINGS FROM TIME IMMEMORIAL

○

The earliest forms of life are said to have emerged from clay. The ancients believed it had generative powers. A myth from ancient China says that Nuwa, a mother-goddess, fashioned the first men out of clay after the world was created. This legend echoes the biblical creation of Adam, who is said to have been born from dust. In both cases, man and earth seem to be at one. . . . Certain deposits, richer or more beautifully colored than others, were more highly prized; thus, Nubian clay was the preferred clay in the ancient Egyptian pharmacopeia. In Greece, Hippocrates prescribed clay dressings for rheumatism, burns, and skin diseases. In China, kaolin—which is used to produce hardy and sparklingly white porcelain—had medicinal uses: its absorption was reputed to cure diarrhea and prevent the progression of cholera. The priest and phytotherapist Sébastian Kneipp brought

"Enjoy the things of the earth
by renouncing them."

GANDHI

its usage back into fashion in the 19th century in the form of poultices and clay-and-vinegar wraps.

ON COLLECTING CLAY

Natural clay soils solidify into blocks that are often very hard and compact. The clay is then crushed and purified — or mixed to combine its elements. To preserve its color and quality, it must dry in the sun. So-called superfine and ultra-ventilated clays boast the finest grains. Grains this fine are made into beauty treatments or poultices.

These clays are particularly well suited to dental care and the treatment of the most sensitive skin types.

THE BENEFITS

Bactericidal, antiseptic, and balancing, clay acts gently and encourages cell turnover. It has a healing and softening effect on the skin and hair shafts, which it coats. Porous and absorbent, and also full of beneficial minerals, it acts as blotting paper, carrying away liquids, sebum, and smells. It swaps harmful "ions" and recharges the body.

Moroccan Atlas rhassoul
One of the most celebrated clays, rhassoul, from the word *ghassala*, meaning "to wash" in Arabic, is a volcanic clay soil which can be found in Morocco's vast Atlas Mountains. Its potent absorption and adsorption properties designate it as a remineralizing and revitalizing clay.

French Montmorillon clay
A superfine green clay, dubbed *montmorillonite*, which is made up of fifty percent silica. Rich in mineral salts and trace elements, it is harvested in the quarries of Montmorillon in southern France, and its virtue has been recognized since prehistory. After extraction, it is simply dried in the sun to preserve its minerals and properties. It will cleanse, remineralize, and soothe combination or oily skin.

Ukrainian montmorillonite blue clay
This is one of the rarest clays in the world. Its potency makes it a lifesaver for blemish-prone and damaged skin.

Guadeloupean illite red clay
Red clay is anti-inflammatory; it remineralizes and boosts tired complexions.

Chinese kaolin
The extreme fineness of soft and white kaolinite clay makes it a delight to use. It is imbued with great antibacterial and healing powers.

A FEW PINCHES

Clay masks and baths are universal remedies, which nowadays enable us to offset our deficiencies in certain minerals through transcutaneous absorption. Our increasingly urban lifestyles have separated us from the earth. For thousands of years, men used to coat themselves in mud for protection, and to paint themselves with clay-based ochre paint for show. Thanks to the absorption of minerals by the skin, they thus imbibed beneficial minerals which the body needs in order to function.

Once applied to damp skin, clay must never be allowed to dry fully: any wrap or mask must thus be removed before it hardens completely. Laden with toxins after use, clay cannot be reused and must be discarded. For very sensitive scalps, it can be lightly dusted at the roots of the hair and then carefully brushed, as an alternative to dry shampoos. In order to take full advantage of clay's many virtues, you should select your clay wisely and buy it pure, with no additives, in the form of powder or pressed into slabs. It is recommended to avoid all "ready-to-use" moist preparations. In order to preserve its health benefits and precious ions, clay must not be handled with metal utensils, nor kept in contact with any type of plastic material. It can only be warmed very gently, in a bain-marie. The water that is used to dilute it must be chlorine-free and not heavily mineralized.

"Out of clay, we make a pot,
but it is the emptiness inside which contains what we want."

LAOZI

CLAY-BASED RECIPES

from Officine Universelle

REMINERALIZING CLAY BATH

In the comfort of your bathroom, revel in the benefits and delights of a mud bath, like an elephant in Africa!

Two to three wooden tablespoons of clay can be added to a 97- to 100°F bath—as close to the body's temperature as it gets—in order to turn the clay, in the simplest way imaginable, into a softening, relaxing, toning, or cleansing treatment. To ensure the best possible dissolution of this very fine soil, mix the clay with some warm water in a small ceramic bowl prior to pouring it into the bath, or use a small cotton bag and allow it to infuse the bathwater.

To soften limestone water, for example, and soothe sensitive skin and the skin of young children, white clay works wonders. Red clay gives the bath "toxin-removing" properties, which help you lose weight. Green clay is efficient against fatigue.

PURIFYING FACIAL MASK

A great classic that must be used regularly whenever the epidermis is disrupted, for instance in the spring and fall.

In a ceramic bowl, using a wooden spoon, start by mixing two tablespoons of blue clay with two tablespoons of lavender hydrolate. Once the paste is thoroughly

smooth, apply it to the face, avoiding the eye area. Leave on for ten minutes and rinse with warm, clear water. Pat dry with a spotlessly clean cloth.

RHASSOUL AND HONEY BODY WRAP

A softening and comforting treatment for a Sunday devoted to major cosmetic operations. Commandeer an old sheet and a bunch of old towels to lie down on once you're covered in mud.

Place a fistful of rose petals in a glass measuring cup, fill with simmering water, and allow to infuse for thirty minutes. Filter this decoction and set it aside. Throw away the petals. In a large bowl, using a wooden spoon or a bamboo whisk, mix 2¾ ounces of rhassoul powder with the rose water you just obtained and add five drops of geranium essential oil. Once the resulting paste becomes smooth, add three tablespoons of liquid organic honey. Mix well. Allow the paste to cool down, and apply this wrap to the bust, thighs, stomach, chest, and arms. Lie down in a quiet setting and leave the body wrap on for ten minutes. Rinse with warm water and carefully pat dry.

❖ COCOA ❖

Butter (beans) — Origin: Central America

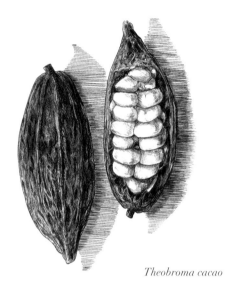

Theobroma cacao

THE TREE
WITH THE GOLDEN FRUIT

◦

Native to Central America, more specifically the Orinoco and Amazon basins, the cocoa tree — whose name simply means "tree" in the Mayan language — is nowadays cultivated in several of the world's tropical regions, where it finds welcome humidity, shade, and heat. It is a delicate tree, grown on small plots in the vicinity of the "*madres del cacao*" — tall trees whose foliage protect it from strong winds and direct sunlight. It is both fragile and prolific; blooming and fruitage occur simultaneously and last all year! The fruit of the cocoa tree, long ovoid berries known as pods, contain dozens of seeds: cocoa beans, whose taste and quality depend on their variety and the local *terroir*. The principal and most famous cocoa varieties are the Forastero (the most rustic and widely cultivated worldwide), the Criollo, and a hybrid of the two, the Trinitario.

TEACHINGS FROM TIME
IMMEMORIAL

◦

Sacred to the Aztecs, this tree was believed to have been a divine gift to the mythical god Quetzalcoatl, who then gave its beans to man. The seeds were used as currency in commercial transactions and to pay taxes. Its presence was recorded in the gardens of the city of Talzipatec, where its cultivation was paired with religious rituals. The *xocohatl* drink, whose natural bitterness was tempered by the addition of honey, fruit, and chiles, was consumed during rites and trances. In 1528, conquistador Hernán Cortés brought chocolate and its uses back to the Spanish court. It quickly became highly prized as a drink. This aristocratic and exotic fad spread to Flanders, which was under Spanish rule at the time, and then slowly on to other European countries. It reached France and Versailles during the reign of Louis XIV. In 1770, Marie-Antoinette arrived at the French court with her own expert, who would earn the title of "Queen's Chocolatier." Swedish botanist Carl Linnaeus nicknamed cocoa *theobroma*, Greek for "food of the gods." With a lower caffeine content than coffee, it contains theobromine, a diuretic and stimulating active ingredient with antidepressant properties. Nevertheless, it was only in the 19th century that cocoa butter started being used in pharmacology, at the time of its relative democratization.

ON COLLECTING COCOA

Cocoa tree pods are harvested twice a year, directly from the branch. They are opened with a cudgel or machete to expose the beans, which are left to ferment in bins for a week, during which time they swell and change color before being laid out to dry. The beans are tossed to ensure even drying, and are then polished either mechanically or by foot. In Trinidad, this stage is known by the pleasant name of "the cocoa dance." Roasting the beans ensures that the cocoa acquires its strong, characteristic taste. They are ground using a millstone to obtain cocoa paste. Once pressed, 2¼ pounds of this paste will yield 1⅔ ounces of cocoa butter (which is an ingredient of chocolate) as well as what is known as cocoa powder. Unrefined cocoa butter is characterized by its deep brown color and its pungent, earthy, and organic aroma.

THE BENEFITS

Made up of palmitic, oleic, and linoleic acids, cocoa butter has nourishing, emollient, stimulating, and regenerative properties. Its theobromine and caffeine content help adipose cells to shrink away. Sterols improve microcirculation, while

"Chocolate is an edible lover."

CASANOVA

polyphenols and vitamin E imbue cocoa with potent antioxidant properties.

HALF A TEASPOON

Cocoa butter is a very dense balm with a pungent smell (some may find it unpleasant; it's a matter of taste): a knob of this butter should be warmed and kneaded between the palms prior to application. Half a teaspoon at most, massaged onto the lips, will provide incomparable protection from the sting of both frost and sun. Regular application on the belly, breasts, and thighs during pregnancy will help reduce the onset of stretch marks. Facial application is highly discouraged for those with acne.

COCOA-BASED RECIPES

from Officine Universelle

UNCTUOUS,
RESTORATIVE BALM

In winter, with the transition to a very dry, unusual climate, the bad habit of biting one's lips during stressful times leaves them in a sorry state.

Avoid all lipsticks until the natural balance of your lips is restored.

In a glass bowl, over a bain-marie, melt two grams of beeswax sheets, three grams of cocoa butter, and five grams of argan oil. Mix using a small glass stirrer, which you have heated beforehand. Once it has become smooth, pour the mixture into a small sterilized jar with a screw-on cap. This will keep for up to a month in the fridge. Massage a small amount of balm onto the lips and the periphery of the mouth before leaving the house every morning, until irritations have disappeared.

Get your triumphant smile back — not to mention the pleasure of soft lips.

FORTIFYING COCOA MASK
FOR STRONG HAIR

Healthy hair will improve its wearer's mood. This mask will be a comfort to both.

In a bowl heated in a bain-marie, melt three to five teaspoons of cocoa butter (depending on the hair's length) and add two to four tablespoons of aloe vera gel; mix thoroughly and let cool. Once the preparation has cooled down, apply to the whole head of hair and wrap in a towel. Leave on for about twenty minutes and follow with a gentle shampoo.

COCOA AND CYPRESS
SLIMMING TREATMENT

Chocolate isn't just a mood lifter: indulge and overindulge in its stimulating properties. In the warmer months, take the time to perform this deliciously scented toning treatment.

Slowly warm 3½ ounces of cocoa butter in a bain-marie until perfectly smooth; add twelve drops of cypress essential oil and five drops of Atlas cedar essential oil. Allow to cool in a lidded glass jar. Once the mixture has cooled down a bit, massage onto the body's affected areas with sustained, deep, upward strokes. This preparation will keep for a month in its jar, tightly sealed, away from direct sunlight.

⌗ COCONUT ⌗

Natural oil pulp — Origin: Philippines and Indonesia

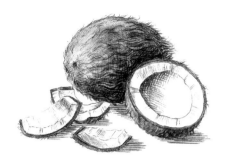

Cocos nucifera

IN THE SHADE OF THE PALMS

○

Whether large or small, the coconut tree, or *Cocos nucifera*, is easily identifiable by its ample and bendy plume of long disheveled fronds. Nowadays, all known species thrive in the inter-tropical area of the globe, especially in coastal regions. Fossilized remains of coconuts dating back several millions of years have been found in India and New Zealand, while fossilized palm fronds have even been excavated in Greenland! The coconut tree spread quickly and naturally, thanks to its perfectly buoyant fruits, which bob from one land to the next following the whims of the currents. Opulent and generous, this resourceful tree produces, depending on its height, nuts of all sizes and shades, and does so for about a hundred years! Within its highly robust shell, in addition to its snowy and nourishing pulp, its fruit contains a refreshing and appetizing liquid: coconut water.

TEACHINGS FROM TIME IMMEMORIAL

○

The coconut has been a lifesaver to sailors and castaways, who used it for both sustenance and drink. Its "trunk"—which in fact is more accurately a stem—is used as construction timber for dwellings and boats. Its leaves make for an admirable roof covering, and its fibers, which surround the fruit's hard shell, are a sturdy material for cordage, baskets, and bags. The inside of the fruit is delicious to the taste, whether fresh or dried. The water held by the fruit is sterile, and—once the nut is opened— keeps rather well. Coconut oil, which oozes forth when the nut is pressed, has been an ingredient of medicinal concoctions and beauty recipes since time began. Monoi oil, for instance, is a deliciously scented maceration of Tiaré and Tamanu flowers in coconut oil.

A LEGENDARY FRUIT

○

In Polynesian mythology, the coconut is omnipresent. One legend centers on a ravishing princess named Hina. Promised by her parents to Faaravaaianuu, she became desperate—as one might imagine—when she found out that her betrothed was in fact a hideous eel! The fair maiden found shelter with the god Maui. After coming out of the lake, her wriggling prince began to chase her, but the protective god captured the hideous beast and then cut it into pieces, only to offer Hina its severed head, wrapped up in a plant-based fabric. "Whatever you do, do not set this package on the ground until you get home, and then plant it at the center of your house's enclosure," the god then recommended. Disregarding this piece of advice, Hina set her package down along the way to go for a swim. The earth then split open and swallowed the package. A plant shot up on the spot, soon becoming a tree raised towards the sun: the first coconut tree! Hina remained at its foot to keep watch over this new resource. Days passed, a drought came, and only the coconut tree was able to resist. Everyone's hunger and thirst was then quenched by the meat and water held in the fruit of this miraculous tree, which had become a literal lifesaver.

ON COLLECTING COCONUT OIL

The traditional extraction process of coconut oil involves harvesting and crushing the fruit's meat, and then pouring it into a gauze-covered piece of wickerwork. Water is then added to this pulp, which is patiently kneaded. The oil rises to the surface; it is collected and gently heated so as to remove all traces of water. The nut is made up of 62 to 65% oil, and just 6% water. Nowadays, the most widespread production method consists of the centrifugation of coconut milk. Copra oil is another variant, for which the pulp is dried before it is pressed and refined. Traditional virgin coconut oil can be identified by its limpidity and light, fresh coconut scent. This oil solidifies naturally below 75°F.

THE BENEFITS

Made up of close to 50% lauric acid, a decongestant and antiparasitic fatty acid, this oil is especially well absorbed by the skin and hair. As for myristic acid, also present in high concentration, it has cleaning and purifying properties. Caprylic and capric acids help soothe the skin thanks to their antibacterial and antifungal properties. Vitamin A speeds up cell turnover and enhances the skin's appearance, while vitamin E protects against oxidation.

A FEW DROPS

A few drops of coconut oil on a damp, warm cotton pad make for a magnificent makeup remover. In winter, solidified coconut oil is an excellent lip balm, which can be dabbed on with the tip of a finger, much like a solid perfume! In summer, coconut oil is ideal for nourishing parched hair that has been weakened by repeated swims and lengthy sunbaths. Coconut milk is a perfect everyday hair treatment to get rid of dry ends.

COCONUT-BASED RECIPES

from Officine Universelle

COCONUT AND SUGAR BODY SCRUB

On select Sundays, instead of launching into making one too many desserts, take a few minutes to whip up this exfoliating, deliciously scented mixture.

To cover the whole body, in a metal bowl mix five tablespoons of coconut oil, seven tablespoons of brown sugar (unrefined or otherwise), and a tablespoon of warm water (or rose hydrolate for extra luxuriousness). Apply in your bathtub while sitting, so as not slip. Patiently scrub the entire body, then rinse with warm water.

With such soft skin, you'll be the most appealing candy!

INSTANT TONE-BRIGHTENING MASK

If you're lucky enough to find a fresh coconut in the vicinity of your deck chair, get to making this skin-care concoction. White lily macerate can be replaced with another complexion-improving oil, such as peach kernel oil.

Blend together four tablespoons of fresh coconut pulp, one teaspoon of white lily macerate, and one teaspoon of organic honey. Apply the resulting paste to the face, avoiding the eye area.

The effect of certain skin treatments is often enhanced by sipping an exotic cocktail!

"It is the fate of a coconut husk to float, for the stone to sink."

MALAWIAN PROVERB

⟡ COPAIBA ⟡

Oil, essential oil (resin) — Origin: Amazonia

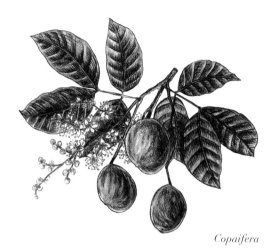

Copaifera

THE JESUIT BALM

◦

In the humid forests of Brazil and Colombia, in Peru and Venezuela, the copaiba stands tall over the canopy with all the might of its massive, short-limbed trunk. The tree is easy to locate due to the pungent smell of its rugged bark, from which flows a precious and curative oleoresin that amazes researchers to this day with its potency and worth. The tree's green leaves shine brightly, and its heartwood is used in carpentry and naval construction. Although several species coexist within the *Copaifera* genus, they all have the same properties: the Amazonian *reticulata*, the Mexican, Caribbean, and tropical African *officinalis*. . . . The tree from which the cosmetic natural oil is most commonly extracted is the *Copaifera langsdorffii.*

TEACHINGS FROM TIME IMMEMORIAL

◦

This tree is a symbol of vitality for Amazonian peoples. Its name, *kupai'wa*, means "there is something inside." It is said that the peoples of the forest began using the *copaibeiras* therapeutically when they saw animals which were wounded or suffering from a poisonous bite rub themselves against its bark. The oil has traditionally been used to strengthen the immune system and to ease digestion. The *curanderos* — healers — have long been applying it as an ointment to heal war injuries and collision wounds and to soothe aching joints. In Panama, copaiba oil was ritually given to newborns with a little bit of honey to chase away evil spirits and develop the child's knowledge of the world. One of the first missionaries in Brazil, Jesuit José de Anchieta, wrote of the copaiba in his long letter to the Superior General of his order in the late 1560s: "It exudes a very pungent smell, but it has a great capacity to help wounds scar over, in such a way that sooner or later no scar remains at all."

As early as the 18th century, its properties were mentioned in the universal dictionary of medicine: "As regards copaiba balm, it is universally esteemed: it will heal any fistula, no matter how old."

ON COLLECTING COPAIBA OIL

○

The copaiba's oleoresin is collected by directly incising and drilling through the bark, much like with maple syrup. Only relatively old trees, those around a hundred years of age, can be used, because that is when they start producing greater quantities of oleoresin. Local populations used to collect this oil only once a year as part of a ceremony. One tree will yield about 10½ gallons per year. The incision made in the trunk is later sealed — preferably with clay — and it takes the tree six months to replenish its oleoresin supply, shielded from the assaults of insects and spores. This method of harvest, patient and respectful, is fortunately still in use, along with another, more invasive and destructive method, which involves hacking away at the trunk with an ax in different spots. . . . The tree is then unproductive for several years. The tint of the collected oleoresin varies from yellow to brown, depending on the resin and essential oil content (between 30 and 90% for the latter). Its aroma is strong, resinous, and woody. It is filtered a number of times and distilled to separate the wholesome vegetable oil from the high-quality essential oil.

THE BENEFITS

○

Copaiba balm is so powerful it is often nicknamed the forest's antibiotic. The beta-caryophyllene concentrated in the oil is anti-inflammatory and antispasmodic. Vitamin E helps cells fight oxidation. Germacrene D has major antibacterial and antifungal properties. Oleic acid (omega-9) helps injuries scar over, while linoleic acid (omega-6) assists cell regeneration and prevents drying. Copaiba oil soothes acne, reduces wrinkles, moderates imbalances and psoriasis, alleviates calluses, takes care of bruises, and soothes sunburn and irritations.

A FEW DROPS

Copaiba oil is a panacea of the forest; topical application has numerous uses. Applying a few drops to the face every night after removing all traces of makeup will work wonders on mature as well as young skin. Beware not to ingest it, though — it's toxic in high doses.

"There is no need to travel round the world and cross oceans and jungles to experience the charms of clouds, the sap of trees, the language of rivers and nights."

JOSEPH KESSEL, *Des hommes*

COPAIBA-BASED RECIPES
from Officine Universelle

RELAXING MASSAGE
AFTER EXERCISE

Hurray for sports! Keep it right up — don't let muscle stiffness drag you down. There is a balm for everything, this included!

In a small bowl, mix one tablespoon of copaiba oil with two tablespoons of shea butter, which you will have warmed between your palms until malleable. This balm must be massaged deeply into your arms, thighs, and muscles after a shower or bath.

ANTI-CALLUS SERUM

Who could possibly teach us more about the art and importance of walking barefoot than the indigenous peoples of Amazonia? Follow in the footsteps of the Guarani warriors.

In a small one-ounce jar with a dropper, mix ten drops of palmarosa essential oil with five drops of eucalyptus essential oil, and fill the remainder with copaiba oil. Apply every night to freshly cleansed and dried feet, massaging the calloused areas.

"FAREWELL BLEMISHES"
BALM

A minor disappointment was lurking in your mirror this morning: your peachy complexion is sporting a blemish. Quickly apply this miracle balm and your morale won't even have the time to suffer. . . .

In a small two-ounce jar with a dropper, mix one part copaiba oil, one part carrot macerate, and one part wheat bran oil with five drops of tea tree essential oil. A few drops on the face every night after gentle but meticulous cleansing will soothe young skin and alleviate the discomfort caused by acne.

✤ CORN POPPY ✤

Flowers and petals — Origin: Europe and North Africa

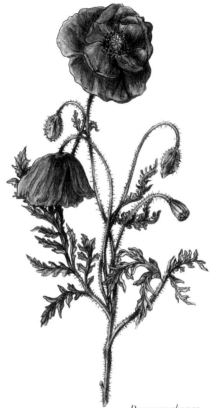

Papaver rhoeas

COQUELICOT

This sylphlike flower with its four scarlet petals, often seen dancing along country lanes, gets its French name from the cockerel's crest, and recalls the bird's cry: *coquelicot, cocorico. . . .* This wildflower used to mingle with grains in the fields, as some of its English and German names ("field poppy" and *Feldmohn*) indicate. Its longevity is due to the hardiness of its seeds, which can survive underground without germinating for extended periods of time. . . . Once the soil is turned over, with a little help from the air and sun, corn poppies will quickly spring up all over the place! Today, this cousin of the opium poppy, often wiped out by the horrendous herbicides of standardized agriculture, timidly lets the trembling silk of its petals fly in the breeze on the edge of the fields. . . .

> *"The sunset has donned
> its poppy cloth,
> It relishes this elegant color
> on its cheeks."*

IBN ATEYA IBN AZZÂQQÂQ

TEACHINGS
FROM TIME IMMEMORIAL
◦

Legend has it that the Arab/Andalusian prince Annou-Mâne ordered the protection of this pretty flower after a wreath of poppies, grasses, and nearby plants was swiftly woven for him as a shield against the sun's rays. In Europe, the soothing properties of the poppy have always been known. The Celts mixed a measure of its sap into their infants' gruel to get them to sleep. Its infusion has a calming effect on nervous people. Trévoux's *Dictionary* (written 1704–71), states that "this plant's flowers are placatory and apt to make the patient spit during fluxions of the chest, common colds and dry coughs." Its incandescent red hue dazzles the eye, but the shine fades away as soon as the flower is plucked. In the 18th century, red blushes were in fashion and women used to craft their own "ponceau ribbons," made from silk or crepe paper, and reddened with the poppy's pigment. Applying such a ribbon (moistened with a little water) to the cheeks would boost their color. The *aker fassi*, that famed and ancient Berber rouge, is a small earthenware disc that is dipped into a pomegranate-peel-and-poppy bath. After the surface has been moistened, it can be applied to the lips or cheekbones with a finger or a brush.

ON COLLECTING POPPIES
◦

Cultivated in Morocco and Albania, poppies are harvested in the spring, and their petals are left to macerate in a mixture of water and alcohol so as to extract the active agents that they contain.

THE BENEFITS
◦

Rhoeadine brings its soothing properties to corn poppy–based preparations. High concentrations of mucilage (botanic polysaccharides) soften and hydrate the skin. The corn poppy owes its ravishing color to anthocyanocide pigments, which are excellent antioxidants—much like the flavonols and flavones that it also contains in abundance.

A FEW PETALS

A generous fistful of corn poppy petals can be thrown under the stream of hot water as you draw yourself a bath and left to infuse for about ten minutes. Diving into this colorful, soothing bath means leaving it with renewed calm and a rosy complexion. The plant must not be eaten, nor should its infusion be drunk, as both carry a risk of intoxication.

⊹ CORNFLOWER ⊹

Hydrolate (flower) — Origin: Middle East

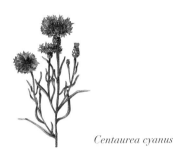

Centaurea cyanus

THE BELLE OF THE HARVEST

○

The cornflower, *Centaurea cyanus*, is common in Europe and thrives from springtime to late summer on the edges of wheat fields and along country lanes, in friendly cohabitation with the poppy. Simultaneously modest and renowned, the cornflower spreads cheer far and wide, from Marie-Antoinette's Sèvres porcelain service to Claude Monet's paintings, thanks to its star-shaped serrated petals and their dazzling mauve-blue pigmentation. It is also known as "hurtsickle," "bluebottle," "bachelor's button," and "boutonniere flower." Chemical weedkillers used in agriculture have chased it away from the field and into the garden, where it is celebrated for its vivacity and pastoral charm.

TEACHINGS FROM TIME IMMEMORIAL

○

Its Latin name is an homage to the healing centaur and herbalist Chiron who, as legend has it, passed on his knowledge to the Greek hero Achilles, whom he taught and healed. The flower's properties and its beauty have been celebrated since ancient times: archeologists found a cornflower crown on Tutankhamun's mummy when his sarcophagus was opened. In the 16th century, herbalist Pierandrea Mattioli recommended the plant as a remedy for eye troubles, by color analogy. . . . Since then, it has been recommended to wash one's eyes with an infusion of the flowers, or to apply this fluid to the eyelids using a compress so as to minimize ophthalmic fatigue. The petals can also be used as poultices. The plant's properties have been clearly established in modern times.

ON COLLECTING CORNFLOWER HYDROLATE

○

The flowers are harvested as soon as they bloom so that they can be distilled. This so-called "noble" distillation produces cornflower hydrolate but no essential oil. Its scent is reminiscent of fresh grass.

THE BENEFITS

○

Pectin and polyyne give the flower its anti-inflammatory, astringent, and decongesting properties, which notably work wonders on the thin skin of the eyelids.

A FEW DROPS

A daily spray of cornflower hydrolate over the entire face soothes the skin after thorough cleansing. Compresses soaked with cornflower hydrolate will efficiently relieve tired and irritated eyes, and revive uneven and lifeless complexions.

CORNFLOWER-BASED RECIPES
from Officine Universelle

SMOOTHING, DECONGESTING MASK

This extremely soft clay-based mask restores balance to sensitive skin.

In a small bowl, carefully mix half a tablespoon of cornflower hydrolate with one tablespoon of pink clay. Apply on the face and the area around the eyes (without getting too close!), avoiding the upper eyelids. Leave on for ten minutes, then rinse with fresh water. Finish by spraying the face with some hydrolate and applying your favorite facial oil.

TONING FACIAL LOTION

Nothing is more simple and efficient than some floral water to gently awaken the skin.

In a small airtight spray bottle, mix one part cornflower hydrolate with one part witch hazel hydrolate and one part rose water. Keep in the fridge for up to two weeks, and spray on your face to give your complexion a radiant boost.

You may also try your own combinations, depending on your skin type.

"A cornflower is out of place in a field of wheat, yet who can deny that the latter owes the former its splendor?"

CONSTANTŸN HUYGEN

❖ DAISY ❖

Macerate (flowers) — Origin: Europe

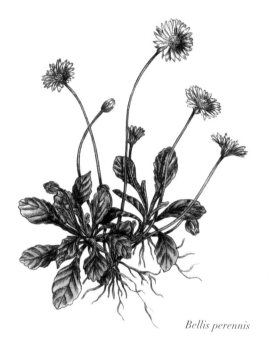

Bellis perennis

TEACHINGS FROM TIME IMMEMORIAL

ₒ

A symbol of innocence, youth, and purity, the daisy adorned the coat of arms of Louis IX, King of France. In the Middle Ages, Gerard of Cremona, an Italian translator of Greek and Arabic scientific books, recommended crushing the flower in some fresh butter as a way to treat joint pain. From the 15th and 16th centuries onward, it was used in poultices to heal bruises. Popular wisdom advocates eating the first three daisy flowers of the year to avoid toothaches.

ON COLLECTING DAISY FLOWERS

ₒ

In the springtime, far from all pollution, the daisy flowers are harvested and put out to dry—but they don't lose all their moisture. In a jar that must be left open for the duration of this first maceration, these flower tops are steeped in a fine, neutral vegetable oil. This preparation is left to macerate for a month, exposed to sunlight but not left directly under its rays. It is then filtered and decanted to rid the macerate of any trace of moisture, which could oxidize and contaminate the preparation.

THE DAY'S EYE

ₒ

At dawn, this adorable little plant, which decorates domesticated lawns and wild prairies alike, turns its bright yellow heart and pinkish-white crown of petals towards the sun. This "day's eye"—hence "daisy"—folds its beautiful limbs by nightfall, or in the event of inclement weather. The daisy plays a role in Celtic myths and legends. An "eternal beauty," as the Latin name promises, it blossoms on warm days (around Easter, in the spring!) and returns every year, perennially pretty—thus symbolizing the comforting hope of life's eternal return.

THE BENEFITS

Daisy macerate is reputed to efficiently tone and tighten the outline of the face, the neck, and the neckline area. The beta-myrcene that it contains decongests and stimulates the skin. Vitamin A activates cell turnover and bioflavonoids stimulate microcirculation. Its antibacterial and antifungal properties are courtesy of its polyacetylenes and triterpenoids.

A FEW DROPS

Daisy macerate is a perfect gift for young mothers who are watching their figure and for all who aim to maintain the freshness and radiance of their cleavage. It should be massaged directly onto the skin.

DAISY-BASED RECIPES
from Officine Universelle

TONING TREATMENT FOR THE FACE, NECK, AND NECKLINE AREA

An irresistible treatment to firm up your contours and curves, from forehead to cleavage, as your thoughts drift back to spring.

In a small jar with a dropper, mix two tablespoons of daisy macerate, two teaspoons of rose hip seed oil, and two teaspoons of prickly pear oil. Use this serum nightly, at bedtime, on gently yet meticulously cleansed skin.

THE ODALISQUE'S OIL— "DOWN WITH HAIRS AND FAT DIMPLES!"

Even if you're perfectly at ease with nudity, both on the beach and in the city, you would still understandably want to fight these perfectly natural imperfections. . . . Serious types will opt for this treatment all year long, while the rest of us will settle simply for summer use.

In a four-ounce jar with a dropper, mix one part daisy macerate and one part nut grass oil with ten drops of Atlas cedar essential oil and five of Mediterranean cypress.

✤ EVENING PRIMROSE ✤

Oil (seeds) — Origin: North America

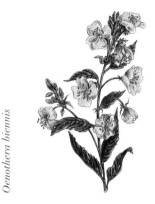

Oenothera biennis

ROYAL MEDICINE

T he evening primrose is a New World lady of the night. It belongs to the family of Onagraceae, which includes several other species. The yellow flowers of the evening primrose open up at sunset, exhaling a fragrance that inebriates nocturnal butterflies. Thriving in the wild on embankments and dunes, the flowers of the evening primrose conquered Europe in the 18th century, thanks to their seeds that crossed the Atlantic as stowaways on American ships, earning the title of "King's cure-all" in England.

TEACHINGS FROM TIME IMMEMORIAL

Legend has it that an infusion of evening primrose flowers makes it possible to tame wild beasts. Amerindian hunters rubbed this infusion on their shoes to make it easier to approach their prey. They consumed its roots and seeds. The plant was reputed to reduce inflammation and ease skin ailments. Infusions of its leaves and flowers were said to help alleviate sore throats.

ON COLLECTING EVENING PRIMROSE OIL

Flowering from June to September, the evening primrose produces tiny brown seeds that are harvested and left to dry so as to increase their concentration in precious omega-6 fatty acids. Later, they are cold-pressed in order to preserve the fragile polyunsaturated fatty acids they contain. Some add vitamin E (tocopherol) to this oil to protect it from oxidation.

THE BENEFITS

Evening primrose oil is made up almost exclusively of unsaturated fatty acids. Rich in gamma-linoleic acid (omega-6), it fosters the production of a hormone that inhibits inflammatory processes and helps alleviate premenstrual syndrome. These phytosterols and triterpenes have restorative, healing, anti-inflammatory, and antioxidant properties. Together, they activate microcirculation, slow down skin aging, and protect from UV damage.

JUST A FEW DROPS

Evening primrose oil is the go-to feminine treatment for time-tested mature and dehydrated skin. Premenstrual breast tenderness can be alleviated by a massage with evening primrose oil. Applying a few drops to the face every night after makeup removal works wonders on everyone and all skin types. It may also be time for you to try eating some flowers! Just sprinkle salads with the delicate and rich yellow flowers of the evening primrose.

EVENING PRIMROSE–BASED RECIPES

from Officine Universelle

FRESH COMPLEXION
TREATMENT OIL

You're never too old to sport a fresh complexion! This treatment should be performed daily in the morning by applying a few drops on damp skin when leaving the shower, just before you enjoy your cup of tea. Before slipping into your clothes, allow yourself one glance in the mirror and witness, with a sigh of relief, that your skin isn't shiny. It's absorbed everything!

In a two-ounce jar with a dropper, mix two teaspoons of evening primrose oil and two teaspoons of rose hip seed oil with five drops of rose geranium essential oil. Apply to the face and neck each morning or night, depending on your preferences and habits.

"FAREWELL SORROWS"
AROMATIC BATH

Life isn't fair, and your body is a stark reminder of that. Time for a good bath! Don't underestimate the beneficial power of warm water infused with the proper ingredients.

In a bowl, whisk together two teaspoons of evening primrose oil with three tablespoons of Epsom salts (high in magnesium), and two drops of clary sage essential oil. Pour this mixture under a stream of warm water in a bath that is already half-full. Wait three minutes to let it infuse, remaining close to the exhalations of the essential oil, which are good for you. A ten-minute soak will get you back on your feet. When you get out of the bath, wrap yourself up in a warm bathrobe and lie down for about ten minutes, taking deep breaths.

⬥ GERANIUM ⬥

Hydrolate, essential oil (flowers, leaves, stems) — Origin: South Africa

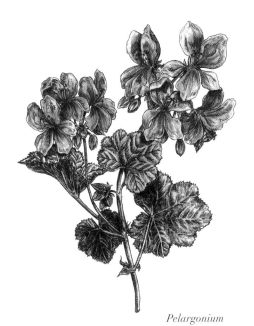

Pelargonium

THE POSSIBILITY OF A ROSE

○

There are several varieties of aromatic geraniums, such as *Pelargonium tomentosum*, with its minty fragrance, and *Pelargonium odoratissimum* and its apple notes. But the most famous one is known as rose geranium, a pelargonium with highly serrated leaves, which originates from South Africa and, as the name indicates, exudes a rose-like fragrance. Pelargonium has a real knack for mimicking other scents. . . . Its leaves and flowers are highly prized by perfumers because of their lemony, spicy notes, enhanced by a touch of sweetness. This simultaneously lively and complex aroma makes it the perfect ally of the rose, whose scents are sometimes very similar. In the mid-19th century, the scarcity of the Damask rose led perfumers to seek other flowers with similar aromatic profiles. The rose geranium, whose moniker testifies to this origin story, was acclimatized on the island of La Réunion and in North Africa; its distillation and use became more prevalent at the end of the century.

TEACHINGS FROM TIME IMMEMORIAL

○

The name, derived from the Greek *geranos* – "crane" – was reportedly inspired by the shape of the geranium's fruit, which the ancients found reminiscent of a crane's beak. Planting a geranium in front of a house is reputed to protect it; in the Piedmont of Italy region, front-door locks are rubbed with the sap of its leaves, so as to secure the home's entrance and keep out intruders! The plant is recognized around the world for its hemostatic and antiseptic properties. Its fragrance induces euphoria, restores vigor, and bolsters willpower. Because of its ability to drive away insects and pests, it has become a go-to addition to balconies, windowsills, and terraces, which it perfumes throughout the summer, all the while ensuring peace and quiet. . . . A few dried leaves will lend a pleasant fragrance to linens, and a few more, infused into herbal tea, will enhance many a dessert or a syrup.

> *"Never trust a man or woman who does not have a passion for geraniums."*

B. NICHOLS-M.HALL

ON COLLECTING GERANIUM HYDROLATE AND ESSENTIAL OIL

Distillation is a subtle art. The essence of the geranium is secreted by hairs that grow on the leaves and stems. In order to extract the full measure of the geranium's potent, fragrant essence, its fresh leaves, flowers, and stems are placed on the grate of an alchemical still and exposed to a flow of water vapor, which carries the aromatic molecules away. This vapor then cools down in a so-called worm condenser and condenses: the hydrolate and the essential oil separate.

THE BENEFITS

Hemostatic, healing, and antiseptic, geranium hydrolate treats oily and acne-ridden skin types, as well as dull complexions. The terpene ester it contains alleviates micro-inflammation and soothes skin irritations. Sesquiterpenes foster cell turnover. Geranium essential oil can be used pure on a small cut. Diluted down to 20% in a neutral, natural vegetable oil, it's soothing and comforting to both the epidermis (thanks to its effect on sensitized skin) and the soul (thanks to its aroma).

A FEW DROPS

Purifying and astringent, the hydrolate can be applied with a cotton pad as a toner to awaken dulled complexions and soothe the discomfort of acne. Refreshing and soothing, it makes for an effective aftershave treatment, which can be complemented by one or two drops of pomegranate oil to maximize its effect. Rose geranium hydrolate will also efficiently complement the natural deodorizing action of alum stone, which regulates excessive perspiration. The pleasant aroma of rose geranium hydrolate and essential oil, which improves and balances the mood, is surely an additional benefit that comes with using it—it is so enjoyable that a certain amount can be added to many facial and body care concoctions, both for its toning properties and its fragrance.

GERANIUM-BASED RECIPES

from Officine Universelle

QUICK! MY SALTS!

You no longer wear a corset; you do not faint easily and you can usually keep your emotions under control. But today, in the privacy of your bathroom, you find yourself at the end of your tether, and it is time to calm down. The choice of background music is up to you, but it is up to us to insist on the soothing virtues of geranium.

If you are lucky enough to have a fragrant geranium plant on your balcony, select twenty leaves and cut them into flakes. What comes next may remind you of the recipe for a famous cocktail, and give you ideas for your next party. Place the leaves in a mortar with two ounces of sea salt and a scant tablespoon of rose water.* Crush with great care so as to extract the geranium's essence. Pour into a hot bath, splash around, and forget about it all.

Non-gardeners are also entitled to some peace of mind: simply add five drops of rose geranium essential oil to two ounces of sea salt, mix, and pour into your bath.

CALMING LOTION
FOR BLEMISH-PRONE SKIN

A bit of softness and firmness to restore some tone and balance to the skin. Antiseptic and anti-inflammatory, this lotion decongests the complexion and perfects facial cleansing.

In a spray bottle, mix one part rose geranium hydrolate with one part rosemary hydrolate. Keep this lotion in the fridge. In the morning, its freshness will smooth out your complexion. Dip a cotton ball into this mixture along with three drops of nigella oil to turn it into an effective nightly cleanser.

Keep in mind that blemish- and acne-prone skin types are often sensitive and off-balance. One should treat them with a gentle touch, and refrain from damaging them further with astringent products or harsh scrubs.

SOOTHING SELF-MASSAGE

In Asia, self-massage is a common and simple practice, which you too can adopt as a habit at the end of a long day.

Add one or two drops of rose geranium essential oil to one tablespoon of marula oil, then indulge in a relaxing massage, from your lower back to the nape of your neck and your shoulders.

This light, fragrant oil alleviates the effects of stress and gives a boost to low spirits.

⊹ GINKGO BILOBA ⊹

Powder and hydrolate (leaves) — Origin: World

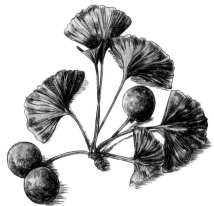

Ginkgo biloba

THE MILLION-YEAR
MAIDENHAIR TREE

◦

This surprising dioecious (all-male or all-female) conifer, with splendid fan-shaped flat leaves, belongs to the oldest family of trees on Earth. Ginkgos have been around for more than three hundred million years, and their fossils have been found all over the globe. However, only a single species survived the particularly violent planetary and climatic shifts at the end of the Primary (or Paleozoic) era: *Ginkgo biloba*, which prudently retreated to the humid forests of present-day China, and from there to Japan and Korea. Its life span can well exceed a thousand years, and it has no known parasites or diseases. Its longevity and resilience in the face of pollution have greatly contributed to its fame, in particular after the dreadful nuclear bombing of Hiroshima—the *Ginkgo biloba* was the first tree to be reborn on the desolate site, less

than a kilometer from ground zero. . . . As a matter of fact, monks have always planted the tree close to their temples to ward off the ravages of fire. The ginkgo was introduced to Europe in the 18th century for the elegance of its bearing and its lobed leaves, which take on a radiant yellow color in the fall. The graceful contours of this leaf inspired Asian artists and were channeled into the hairstyles of the fair ladies and samurais of the Edo period. The shape was later beautifully reborn under the paintbrushes and chisels of the Western masters of art nouveau and the Craftsman movement.

TEACHINGS FROM TIME
IMMEMORIAL

◦

"Ginkgo" is the transcription of a Chinese ideogram meaning "silver apricot." "Biloba" was added by Carl Linnaeus in 1771 as a reference to the dual lobe of its leaves. Traditional Chinese medicine makes use of the female tree's seeds, which are contained in a particularly malodorous fruit; the kernel forms part of many treatments that fight asthma and other respiratory ailments. The Chinese medical treatise *Shen Nung Pen T'sao Ching* is the first work that mentions its blood flow–boosting properties. In the 15th century, the *Dian Nan Ben Cao*, a medicinal herbarium, mentions the use of ginkgo leaves in skincare and combating freckles. Since the 1932 discovery of ginkgolides (one of its components) and their use in Western medicine, the tree has been grown everywhere. This enables the production of treatments that alleviate circulatory problems and boost memory—the ginkgo has a high concentration of potent antioxidants with neuroprotective properties.

antioxidant properties, which are far superior to   those of, for example, vitamins C and E. They bind with collagen and help preserve the structure of tissues. Highly concentrated ginkgolides and terpene lactones boost circulation.

A FEW DROPS

Ginkgo hydrolate can be applied to the body every morning as a seasonal cure to invigorate the network of capillaries, those tiny surface blood vessels. Ginkgo powder, which is used in many dietary supplements reputed to ward off memory loss, is also an interesting ingredient to add to your masks (aim for a proportion of gingko of about 10% of the total). Ginkgo leaves are also natural insecticides, and can be inserted protectively between the pages of old books.

ON COLLECTING
GINKGO BILOBA

Ginkgo biloba leaves are harvested when they are just starting to turn yellow; they are then put out to dry and crushed to a powder. Hydrodistillation also allows for the production of a ginkgo leaf hydrolate. Seeds can be eaten like pistachios and are said to be an aphrodisiac. . . .

THE BENEFIT

When it comes to aging well, *Ginkgo biloba* is your best ally. The oligo-proanthocyanidins—flavonoids—in its leaves have remarkable

"Treading on the Ginkgo's golden leaves
The child leisurely
Comes down the mountain"

Yosa Buson (1716–83)

GINGKO BILOBA–BASED RECIPES

from Officine Universelle

BALANCING CLEANSING PASTE

Forget for an evening the automatic resort to cotton pads and lotions. Your skin deserves the best, and do not think that cleansing means stripping. This oxygenizing ritual should be performed once or twice a week.

Pour one tablespoon of ginkgo powder and two teaspoons of kaolin clay into a non-metallic container and mix with a wooden spatula. Soften a tablespoon of shea butter in a bain-marie and carefully blend it with the dry ingredients. Massage onto the face: start with the sides of your nose, working your way outwards; focus on the chin and finish with the temples and forehead using gentle, circular motions. Rinse with copious amounts of water.

Do not rush this: a gentle facial cleansing massage bestows numerous benefits on skin tone and appearance. Take your time; breathe in, breathe out. You may then finish by moisturizing your cleansed, freshened skin.

GINKGO-BASED
ETERNAL BEAUTY MASK

Caring for the face and neck area is something that must be done regularly, but without excess or obsession. This is a mask that can be applied once a week to greatly enhance your complexion.

In a small bowl, using a bamboo whisk, carefully mix one tablespoon of ginkgo hydrolate, one teaspoon of ginkgo powder, one tablespoon of rice bran powder, and one teaspoon of perilla oil. After removing all traces of makeup, apply this smooth paste to your face and neck and leave on for fifteen minutes while reflecting on the bliss of being a part of this world. Rinse with clear water and pat dry with a spotlessly clean cloth.

HEAVY LEG TREATMENT

Do you feel as if your entire body weight has somehow slumped down to your legs? Stimulate circulation and boost your mood!

In a bowl, carefully mix two teaspoons of ginkgo powder with two tablespoons of aloe vera gel and three drops of Virginian juniper essential oil using a bamboo whisk. Massage with an upwards motion from the calf to around the ankle to the front of the leg and up to the knee. Relief will come instantaneously, but be sure to maximize the effect with five minutes of exertion: lie down on your back, breathe slowly, raise your legs (keeping them straight) perpendicular to your back, and draw circles in the air with your feet.

⟡ GRAPE ⟡

Oil (seeds) — Origin: Caucasus

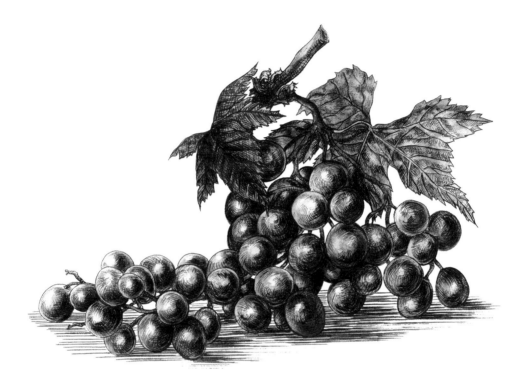

Vitis vinifera

THE VINE'S TENDRILS

Vitis vinifera is a very hardy fruit tree that can live past one hundred: its resilience is legendary and outstanding, even in harsh climatic conditions and on poor soils. Viticulture is one of the oldest forms of cultivation practiced by mankind. The wild vine, a liana of sylvan origins, acclimatized throughout Europe and the Mediterranean basin. Its cultivation for wine production is said to have originated in the Caucasus, in present-day Georgia, where an ancient winery was discovered. The vine—which is now vastly different from its sylvan ancestor—presently covers over eight million hectares worldwide. Domesticated for its fruit, the grapevine yields other products that keep well: dried grapes, wine, marmalade, and alcohol. France and Italy are the world's foremost wine producers.

TEACHINGS FROM TIME IMMEMORIAL

o

The myth of Dionysus, god of wine, the vine, and the wild, brings to mind the Bacchanalia and the exaltation ("possession by gods") of these wild celebrations, yet he is also a complex god, an intermediary between the world of men and the beyond. Wine is therefore a means of mystical transportation! It is also one of the earliest documented forms of medication. Antiquity's three most famed physicians, Hippocrates, Pedanius Dioscorides, and Claudius Galenus, mention it and document its uses, varieties, and properties. According to Rufus of Ephesus, a Greek physician from the first century AD, "Wine can also put the soul in a certain state, as it is a remedy against sorrow." Wine was also a vehicle for medicinal preparations; it was used in decoctions or to capture and preserve the virtues of plants. In 1652, Nicholas Culpeper, an English herbalist and physician, recommended using the plant as a mouthwash: "the ashes of burnt vine shoots will turn coal-black teeth as white as snow." At the court of the Sun King, wine was used as makeup, to impart a fine complexion. The legendary *eau de charmes*, nicknamed "the tears of the vine," was patiently collected in little vials hanging from the arbors. Its application was said to preserve beauty and a radiant complexion. Nowadays, its proven concentration of antioxidants has inspired vinotherapy, a grape-based regimen of treatments and massages.

ON PREPARING GRAPES

o

Grapes are harvested in September or October, depending on the region, the year and the bunches' degree of maturation. Attempts to extract the thick green oil of grape seeds were made in the early 19th century, but the industrial production of this by-product of viticulture only began in earnest after 1945. Depending on the local climate, grape seeds may contain anywhere from 5 to 20% lipids and essential fatty acids. This oil is usually extracted using a solvent; one should therefore look for varieties which are cold-pressed, which preserves all of its virtues.

THE BENEFITS

o

Black grapes are richer in tannins, vitamins, and minerals than their white counterparts. Their oil contains potent natural active agents: vitamin E is a potent antioxidant, while phenolic compounds help protect cells from oxidation by free radicals. Grapeseed oil is also rich in linoleic acid (omega-6): it protects the skin from external aggressions and efficiently prevents it from drying out. It also helps regulate sebum production.

A FEW DROPS

This beneficial oil deserves to cross over from the kitchen to the bathroom. It is fine-textured, absorbs quickly, and regulates the sebum production of combination and oily skin types, all the while warding off the signs of aging in more mature skin. And of course, from now on, never set aside the seeds when eating grapes: you would miss out on their excellent benefits.

GRAPE-BASED RECIPES
from Officine Universelle

HIGH-RADIANCE MASK

A mask with a spectacular effect, ensuring the freshest appearance and soft, firm skin.

Carefully choose and wash ten black grapes. In a blender, mix them with a teaspoon of grapeseed oil. Apply this mixture to the face and leave on for about ten minutes, then rinse with warm water and pat dry.

"The grape is not ripened by the rays of the moon."

LATIN PROVERB

✣ HEMP ✣

Oil, seeds — Origin: Central Asia

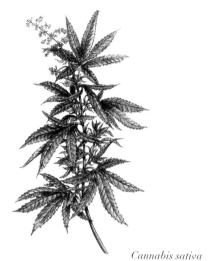

Cannabis sativa

OVER THE HEMP
◦

There's hemp, and then there's hemp. *Cannabis rustica* is the wild plant, whose cultivated varieties are referred to as *sativa*, or textile hemp, in temperate regions, and *indica*, or Indian hemp, in tropical and subtropical regions. The latter variety has flowering tops and its resin has certain psychotropic properties. *Cannabis sativa* is an annual herbaceous plant with serrated leaves, grown throughout the world for its fiber, seeds, and oil. The stem of hemp, whose soft part is known as hemp straw, is made up of very strong fibers, which were once used to make clothing, cordage, and paper. With the rise of cotton and the demise of sailing ships, hemp experienced a drastic decline in Europe. Nowadays, its resilience to disease, the relatively low amount of water

and labor required to cultivate it, its short five-month life cycle, and its numerous potential industrial uses are bringing hemp back into fashion.

TEACHINGS FROM TIME IMMEMORIAL
◦

Hemp was one of the first plants to be cultivated by man. The Greek historian Herodotus described its usage by the Scythes, who placed the seeds on hot stones to serve as incense, intoxicating themselves with its vapors. In Ancient Egypt, the *Ebers papyrus*, one of the world's oldest medical treatises, documents its prescription for soothing contractions during childbirth. Jivaka Khumar Bacha, a traditional physician and friend of the Buddha, used whole hemp leaves to alleviate pain during surgical operations. In China, in the 1st century, the *Shennong Bencaojing* also mentioned it as a remedy against ailments as diverse as gout, rheumatism, constipation, and forgetfulness. In the 14th century, Chinese medicine recommended the consumption of its seeds to ensure longevity and a healthy constitution. In the French countryside, many superstitions were associated with hemp: "You must sing as you're harvesting it, or the weavers will fall asleep while weaving it," "When hens eat hemp seeds, they stop laying eggs and start brooding them . . ."

In his *Treatise on Hemp*, in 1758,
M. Marcandier revealed the customary
therapeutic uses of *Cannabis sativa* oil:
"*Taken as an emulsion, it is effective against
coughs and jaundice. [. . .] The seed and the
green leaves were applied as cataplasms.*"
In his 1826 *Dictionary of Beauty*, César
Gardeton described hemp as a hair
fortifier: "To grow the hair quickly: using
a mortar and pestle, crush any quantity of
hemp stems, which you will sprinkle with
freshly pressed garlic sap."

ON COLLECTING HEMP

When cold-pressed, it yields a green,
herbaceous-scented oil. It is sensitive
to oxidation and should therefore be
refrigerated or used quickly after opening.

THE BENEFITS

Hempseed oil boasts a high concentration
of linoleic acid (omega-6 and omega-3),
which stimulates the epidermis and
helps it fight the damage wrought by free
radicals on the skin. It is soothing and also
calms redness and irritations.

A FEW DROPS

Even though *Cannabis sativa* oil does not
share the hallucinogenic properties of its
Indian cousin, it will efficiently relax tired
and dehydrated skin. It is easy to use, and
daily application will help smooth out
facial features and soothe the epidermis.
It is highly hydrating and will offset
moisture losses.

HEMP-BASED RECIPES

from Officine Universelle

BALANCING OIL

*You practice meditation and running, but in
spite of your dietary efforts, your skin fails
to reflect this lovely inner harmony. Apply
this potent trio nightly, just before bed, to
restore balance. . . .*

In a two-ounce jar with a dropper, mix
one part hempseed oil, one part jojoba oil,
one part grapeseed oil, and add five drops
of palmarosa essential oil—the Indian
geranium.

REVITALIZING BODY OIL

*Daily application of this fine oil will provide
complete satisfaction, with simplicity of
the highest order—improving the look of
blemishes and renewing the skin's firmness
and radiance.*

In a jar with a dropper, mix one part
hempseed oil, one part marula oil, and
one part rosehip seed oil.

⊹ HIBISCUS ⊹

Oil, macerate, flowers (flowers, seeds) — Origin: India

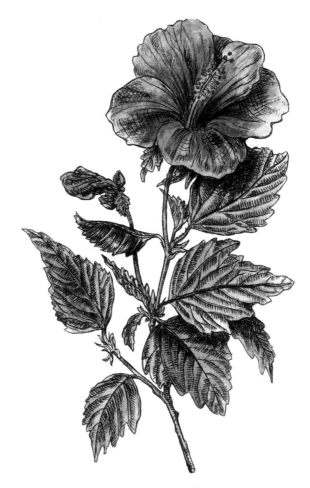

Hibiscus

ETERNITY FLOWERS

○

This island maiden is the flower of Hawaiian surfers, nourishing the paradisiacal archipelagos of our dreams. It is also the national emblem of South Korea and Malaysia, and its Western name comes from the Greek *hibiskos*, a type of mallow. Carl Linnaeus, the famed Swedish naturalist and botanist, gave it this name in his work *Systema Naturae*. This evergreen shrub thrives best in tropical and subtropical regions and numbers more than two hundred varieties, some of which are also edible.

TEACHINGS FROM TIME IMMEMORIAL

In Africa, the purple flowers of the Guinean roselle, *Hibiscus sabdariffa*, lend themselves to numerous culinary preparations, and especially to infusions that improve tonus and digestion, such as the famed Abyssinian pink tea, Senegalese *bissap*, and Egyptian *carcade*. Compresses soaked with a hibiscus flower infusion are reputed to reduce skin inflammation and irritations. The plants' properties are concentrated in its seeds, which yield an oil that is admirably high in vitamins. In India, Ayurveda has long included *Hibiscus rosa-sinensis* (or "China rose") in its precepts, on account of its cosmetic potential. Hibiscus flowers are offered to the gods during the *pujas*—offering rites. In Bengal, hibiscus shrubs are planted in front of houses: their flowers are used to compose garlands to be offered to the gods. The hibiscus—*ardhul* in Hindi or *java kusu* in Sanskrit—is more specifically dedicated to the Indian goddess Kali, or Devi. During the war against the demons, when Mahishasura marched towards paradise at the head of an army of devils, the gods begat the war goddess. But, drunk with fury when she emerged victorious having killed Mahishasura after a terrifying battle, she carried on destroying everything. To stop her, her husband, Shiva, came to the battlefield, where he lay down at her feet to pacify her. Kali kept dancing until she noticed him. Feeling embarrassed, she stuck her tongue out—she is often represented in this manner, and the red hibiscus symbolizes her red tongue, her energy, and her lust for victory. According to other myths, the tree offered its flower to the goddess to make her eyes red with rage. . . . Cultivated in the Middle East and in Asia since antiquity, the hibiscus is decorative and appealing, and has a good medicinal reputation.

ON COLLECTING HIBISCUS

In the countries where the plant thrives, hibiscus flowers are plucked by hand and laid out to dry in the sun. They are then preserved whole, or crushed to a powder that can be used as a dye. In the fall, the flowers' calyxes are harvested and its pods are opened to collect the seeds, which are then cold-pressed to yield a fine, wholesome oil.

THE BENEFITS

High in sugars, in hydrating and softening gum, in trace elements that ensure the efficiency of the skin's enzymatic systems, and in flavonoids that improve microcirculation, hibiscus oil works wonders on both skin tone and hair. It wards off the signs of the passage of time with great efficiency, and is naturally high in vitamin E, which protects cells from oxidation and helps keep the skin smooth and supple. High concentrations of sterols help protect the skin from exposure.

A FEW DROPS

A few drops of hibiscus flower oil are recommended as a topical application to the scalp and full length of the hair, to strengthen and stimulate regrowth.

For any preparation incorporating hibiscus flowers, keep in mind that their coloring power is notorious. Handle with caution.

HIBISCUS-BASED RECIPES

from Officine Universelle

HYDRATING HAIR LOTION FOR COPPER-COLORED VOLUME

This infusion is a rinsing treatment that can be applied as often as desired.

Allow a handful of hibiscus flowers to infuse in one quart of simmering water, away from the heat. Filter the water, and add six tablespoons of rosemary floral water. Adjust the intensity of the red tint depending on the desired result: it is better to start low so as to remain in control of the effect. Guaranteed reddish and coppery shine.

FIERY TREATMENT FOR RADIANT RED HAIR

Someday, to get your color back or to fly it high, try this coloring treatment, which enhances the hair and restores its vigor.

In a bowl, carefully whisk together at least .35 ounces of hibiscus flower powder (depending on the desired intensity), 1¾ ounces of neutral henna, and two tablespoons of sesame oil with a "palmful" of water. Apply section by section, and leave on for thirty minutes.
It is advisable to invest in a plastic cap to put over your hair while the preparation is in place and to protect your shoulders with a cloth whose whiteness can be sacrificed.

⊹ INCA INCHI ⊹

Oil — Origin: Peru

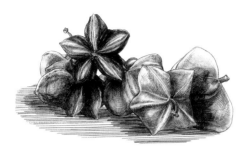

Plukenetia volubilis

THE INCA CHESTNUT!

Plukenetia volubilis is a climbing, star-fruited plant. This "mountain almond" is fond of very supple or even muddy soils, thriving on the edge of forests and, more specifically, at the foot of the Andes. It is cultivated on small, usually family-owned plots. Peru is home to a flora replete with various riches, which often cause envy: "bio-piracy," or the appropriation of traditional resources and knowledge, is widespread, and *Plukenetia volubilis* is a source of great jealousy.

TEACHINGS FROM TIME IMMEMORIAL

The plant has been cultivated for over three thousand years. Its brown seeds, high in proteins, can be eaten roasted and its leaves are eaten cooked. Ceramics from the year 1438, decorated with depictions of the victory of the Incan emperor Pachacuti over the Chankas, show how important the fruits were at the time: they are easily recognizable among the illustrations. In the 16th century, Garcillaso de la Vega, a man of noble Incan lineage on his mother's side and a Spanish aristocrat thanks to his father, shared his idyllic vision of the empire, the Tawantinsuyu, in his book *Comentarios Reales de los Incas*. This included the earliest known description of the plant and its uses.

ON COLLECTING INCA INCHI

The fruit is put out to dry. Once removed from the pulp, the seeds are cold-pressed. The oil is clarified, decanted, and filtered. Approximately eleven pounds of seeds are required to obtain one quart of a delicate oil, with a green, woody scent and a fine, lightweight texture.

THE BENEFITS

Rich in antioxidant components and vitamin E, Inca Inchi oil is a balm for parched skin: it restores the suppleness and comfort of tired or mature skin and generously nourishes younger skin. Its exceptional concentration of linoleic acid (omega-6) and linolenic acid (omega-3) turns it into a veritable shield for the epidermis.

A FEW DROPS

Deliciously fragrant, easy to apply, excellent under all circumstances, Inca Inchi is one of the most remarkable antiaging oils in the world. Its green scent makes it particularly popular among those who dislike the typically earthy aroma of natural oils. The wonderful dry feel is as light as can be. It could easily become the oil you take everywhere: it absorbs quickly and leaves the skin feeling fresh and smooth. It smooths out crumples and enlivens the skin. It also soothes dehydrated combination skin and assuages bouts of rosacea.

INCA INCHI–BASED RECIPES
from Officine Universelle

GREAT AURA MASK

Are you just coming out of the winter, a cold or some other type of crisis? This mask will boost your complexion and make it durably radiant again.

In a small ceramic bowl (so as not to demineralize the clay) mix one tablespoon of Inca Inchi oil, one level tablespoon of red clay, and a scant three tablespoons of rose hydrolate with a bamboo whisk. Whisk until smooth, apply, and leave on for ten minutes. Rinse with clear, warm water and dry without rubbing the skin.

ANTI-ROSACEA SERUM

Is your heart tender and your skin sensitive? Avoid violent temperature swings as well as prolonged sun exposure, and apply this soothing serum.

Fill a small jar with a dropper with two teaspoons of Inca Inchi oil, then add two drops of *Helichrysum italicum* essential oil. Turn the properly closed jar upside down several times, in order to mix without shaking. Apply nightly to clean skin. This mixture will keep for six months to a year.

"The creeper climbs to the top of the tree by clinging to it."

TIBETAN WISDOM

✤ IRIS ✤

Powder (rhizome) — Origin: Italy

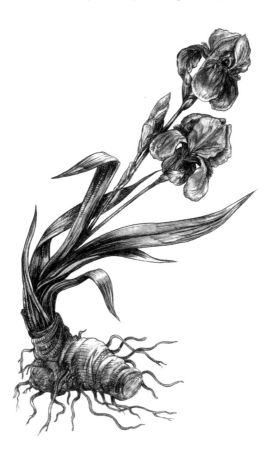

Iris germanica, Iris florentina and Iris pallida

THE FLORENTINE

The iris gets its name from the gods' messenger in Greek mythology, whose shimmering wings left a rainbow in their wake. The elegant Iris was also Hera's chambermaid, and the goddess of fragrance. Boasting a magnificent flower that can be found in every shade, this plant is a rhizome that hails from the Mediterranean basin; it is hardy and easy to cultivate. Shaped like a gladiator sword or a flame, the iris is the flower of Florence, in Tuscany. It was also the emblem of French royalty (an honor that was later usurped by the lily). Legend attributes this choice to Clovis who, during the 507 Battle of Vouillé, having been pursued into a swamp by his Visigoth foes, reportedly hid behind the plant's generous tufts. Victorious and grateful, he is said to have elected to add that lifesaving marshland iris to his coat of arms.

TEACHINGS FROM TIME IMMEMORIAL

❦

The iris exudes a fragrant compound that has been valued since antiquity. The famed 12th-century abbess, healer, and visionary Hildegarde de Bingen recommended its use to alleviate skin conditions: "The iris is dry and warm. Its greenness resides in its root and seeps up to its leaves." A century later, the Bolognese agronomist Pietro de' Crescenzi mentions the cultivation of white and purple irises for medical purposes. Iris was then used to whiten the complexion and clean the teeth. Teething babies were given a piece of iris root to chew on. . . . Upon arriving at the French court, Catherine de' Medici made the iris fashionable as a way to perfume clothes, belts, and gloves. In the 17th century, people would dust their hair with an astringent and fragrant preparation based on iris root powder. To perfume linens, laundrywomen would place iris root in their great batches of laundry in the springtime.

ON PREPARATION

❦

After blooming in May, the flowers are cut so as to strengthen the rhizomes. Once they reach at least three years of age, they are pulled from the earth during the summer and left out to dry in the sun for several days. For cosmetic use, rhizomes are then finely milled and sieved. In perfumery, the roots are left to rest for three to five years before they are used because the concentration in irones, with their characteristic violet scent, increases over time. Iris powder, pale pink in color, exudes a sweet and delicious fragrance.

THE BENEFITS

❦

The gum contained in irises is a natural emollient that hydrates tissues. It is also rich in tannins, which are antioxidant, astringent, and potently antiseptic. As for violine, it has anesthetic and soothing properties.

"I am bored, pluck me some young girls
and blue iris in the shadow of the bowers . . ."

FRANCIS JAMMES, 1898

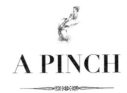

A PINCH

Iris root powder is an ancient remedy to bring radiance to the face and brighten the complexion. Moisten a little iris root powder with some rose water to make a cleansing facial scrub.

One highly aromatic pinch can be added to toothpaste for even cleaner—and whiter—teeth.

IRIS-BASED RECIPES
from Officine Universelle

BRIGHTENING AND BALANCING FACIAL MASK

If you judge your skin solely by the brightness of its complexion and the fineness of its pores, this mask was made for you.

In a small bowl, carefully mix together two tablespoons of iris root powder, one tablespoon of rice bran powder, one tablespoon of geranium hydrolate, and a teaspoon of white lily macerate. This will yield a very supple paste, which can be moistened further depending on the desired texture. Slowly and patiently scrub the face and neckline area with the paste. Rinse, and pat dry with a spotlessly clean cloth.

IRIS PURIFYING BATH

Find inspiration in the purifying tradition of the Japanese iris bath, shobu-yu. *Young children are bathed in it to celebrate their holiday, in May. This bath protects and imparts strength and courage.*

In a very warm bath, scatter the chopped leaves, whole flowers, and sliced roots of three well-cleansed irises. Allow to infuse. After showering (one does not set foot in a treatment bath without having previously rid oneself of impurities), immerse yourself in this bath for five minutes as a family, one person at a time, starting with the youngest.

⟡ JASMINE ⟡

Flower, essential oil, hydrolate — Origin: India

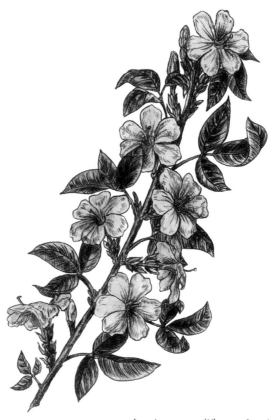

Jasminum grandiflorum, Jasminum sambac

THE ORIENTAL

The starry petals of this flower, centered around a fragrant chalice, are the emblem of Indonesia, Pakistan, and the Philippines. Its Arab name, *yâsamîn*, derives from the Persian *yâsaman*, meaning "white flower." The slender creeping plant originated in the open valleys at the foot of the Himalayas. Florets bloom in bunches at the tip of its stems, like so many umbrellas. There are about two hundred varieties of jasmine, two of which are particularly prized by perfumers and harvesters of "simple" flowers: Arabian jasmine (eight-petaled *Jasminum sambac*) and five-petaled *Jasminum grandiflorum*. As a legendary constituent of high-end perfumes, jasmine has greatly contributed to the fortune of the town of Grasse — the birthplace of the cold *enfleurage* technique, which made it possible to capture its precious scent.

TEACHINGS FROM TIME IMMEMORIAL

◦

The immediately seductive (not to mention sensual) fragrance is reputed to arouse love and pleasure. Legend has it that Cleopatra joined the Roman general Marc Antony aboard a ship whose sails had been soaked in jasmine essence, producing an irresistible breeze . . . "the poop was beaten gold / Purple the sails, and so perfumed that / The winds were love-sick with them," Shakespeare mused. It is said that Kama, the Indian god of love, shot arrows perfumed with jasmine . . . or with blue lotus, mango tree leaf, champak, or shirisha, using his sugarcane bow. As early as the 10th century, in China, jasmine flowers were mixed with green or black tea to dry together. This calming, fragrant tea is reputed to soothe difficult digestion; it also helps with flatulence. Jasmine has been present in Europe since the late 16th century. In Versailles, the plant (imported from Provence) perfumed the court's summer evening promenades and lent its aroma to snuff. Jasmine oil perfumed the "Fargeon-style" ointment which Queen Marie-Antoinette used to care for her hair, stimulate its growth, and prevent it from falling out.

ON COLLECTING JASMINE

◦

This fragile flower, whose scent is as strong as it is hard to capture, is plucked by hand at dawn — or at night in the case of some varieties. Today, in perfumery, alcohol-based extraction (or using some other volatile solvent) is the most commonly used technique to harness the properties of jasmine — first and foremost its perfume. The solvent is then eliminated by evaporation, and a waxy material, the "concrete," is thus isolated. It is then purified by removing the wax and plant residue, yielding the jasmine "absolute."

THE BENEFITS

◦

Jasmine essential oil is relaxing and balancing. Benzyl benzoate, one of its components, is known for its effect on nervous tension and stress; it also helps alleviate depression. Vitamin E, a potent antioxidant, soothes the most sensitive skin types, all the while stimulating them in a positive fashion. It is said that a jasmine tea infusion will also efficiently decongest the area around the eyes.

A FEW DROPS

Prepare an infusion of jasmine flowers to lighten up during periods of anxiety. Stimulate hair growth by massaging their roots with some tamanu oil, enhanced with jasmine absolute — or, better yet, infused with fresh flowers. And perfume the nape of your neck with a veil of *Jasminum sambac* hydrolate to become simply irresistible.

JASMINE-BASED RECIPES
from Officine Universelle

"SUNDAY COMPLEXION" MASK

A Sunday mask to combat the skin's lack of elasticity, and other unwanted signs of aging.

Blend a very fresh, peeled organic carrot. Press out the excess water and add to this pulp one drop of jasmine essential oil and one tablespoon of Inca Inchi oil, and mix well with a fork.

After removing all traces of makeup, apply the resulting paste to the face, avoiding the area around the eyes and lips. Leave on for about ten minutes and rinse with warm water.

"FOLLOW ME" MASSAGE OIL

This scented oil shoos away fatigue and boosts the mood.

In a small two-ounce jar filled with hemp oil, add four drops of jasmine essential oil, four drops of sandalwood essential oil, and three drops of vetiver essential oil. Shake the jar. After showering or bathing, massage this relaxing, attractive oil all over your body.

BRIDAL BATH

Your mind is made up regarding makeup, manicure, and hairstyle, but have you considered the beneficial virtues of a flower bath on both your mood and facial radiance?

In the garden, pluck a few jasmine flowers, rosebuds, and geranium leaves—untreated, of course. Fill a small cotton bag with these flowers and leaves, draw a hot bath, add the bag, and allow it to infuse in the water. Add a glass of orange blossom hydrolate, immerse yourself in this fragrant bath, breathe deeply, and reflect happily on this fine day.

"Happiness is a fragrance which you cannot sprinkle onto others without catching a few drops yourself."

SAINT AUGUSTINE

⬧ JOJOBA ⬧

Oil, wax (seeds) — Origin: Mexico

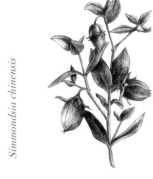

Simmondsia chinensis

Legend has it that the jojoba—or *hohowi* as the locals called it—was a gift from the "Great Spirit," designed to take care of men: it was part of a divinatory drink. Botanist Howard Scott Gentry nicknamed it "Sleeping Princess Jojoba." It elicited interest in the 1930s, but its commercial exploitation only started in the 1970s.

THE MIRAGE TREE

The roots of the jojoba, *Simmondsia chinensis*, dig very deep into the desert floor to find the moisture they need to survive. With its green-colored, blue-haloed leaves, this shrub lives in extreme climatic conditions, enduring of the heat of the high sun and the bite of intense nighttime cold. Its evergreen foliage protects the soil on which it grows. Only the female plants bear nuts, which are eaten by goats and sheep. In the Sonora desert, between Mexico and California, centenary *chohobbas* (their Mexican name) still thrive.

TEACHINGS FROM TIME IMMEMORIAL

In the 1789 *Historia de la Antigua o Baja California*, Jesuit priest Clavijero reports that jojoba was used by the local populations to help wounds scar over, and to heal skin and hair from the effects of the arid climate.

ON COLLECTING JOJOBA OIL

Seeds are harvested five months after the shrub blossoms and are rich in proteins. Tough and ribbed, they are highly resistant and can be pressed long after harvest. They are also generous, containing 45 to 60% oil, and when cold-pressed they yield a yellow wax with a sweet hazelnut scent, whose composition is similar to that of sebum. It has the added merit of not going rancid, and contains few impurities, which enables it to be kept easily and last a long time.

THE BENEFITS

This vegetable wax is composed of a variety of fatty acids (omega-9): gadoleic acid, erucic acid, nervonic acid, and oleic acid, all of which help protect and reinforce the top layer of the epidermis and reduce inflammation. They also contribute to the scarring-over process and help maintain the suppleness of the skin. Palmitic acid increases this softening effect.

A FEW DROPS

Jojoba oil is the best friend of blemish-prone, combination, or oily skin. Too often, people are wary of applying oil to an uneven or oily complexion. In reality, you shouldn't hesitate to do so! A few drops of jojoba oil, regularly applied to the face, will quickly and efficiently normalize sebum production, and thus gently help balance the skin and minimize inflammation. Jojoba is also a perfect makeup remover: a few drops of oil on a cotton pad (doused with water or witch hazel hydrolate) will achieve more than the most sophisticated makeup-removing formulas.

JOJOBA-BASED RECIPES
from Officine Universelle

DRAINING AND REVIVING MASSAGE OIL

Thanks to its light texture, jojoba oil is a fit companion for a massage. Just a few minutes will suffice to ensure its absorption, and your relaxation.

After bathing, mix three tablespoons of jojoba oil with three drops of cypress essential oil in a small bowl. Massage over your whole body, working your way up to the heart, then lie down for ten minutes on a bath towel. Breathe deeply, and turn your thoughts inward.

PURIFYING MASK FOR IRRITATED SCALPS

If you've never experienced oil on your scalp or hair, jojoba oil should be your first choice. It is as easy to use as it is to rinse off, which makes it an appealing and practical option.

In a bowl, using a bamboo whisk, carefully mix one tablespoon of healing and anti-inflammatory jojoba oil with an egg yolk and—for enjoyment's sake—two drops of ylang ylang, palmarosa, or rose geranium essential oil.

KALAHARI MELON

Oil (seeds) — Origin: Namibia

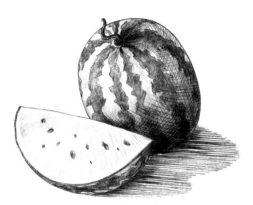

Citrullus lanatus

THE WILD WATERMELON

Even though the shape of the famed Kalahari melon is reminiscent of our sweet watermelon, its pale yellow or green pulp is very bitter. The only connections it has to its distant cousin are its appearance and botanical proximity. Its cultivation reportedly started in the Nile Valley in the centuries predating the start of history; today there are four species of this melon in tropical and subtropical Africa, including one that thrives in the scrubby desert plains of the Kalahari, a very dry savanna that stretches from Botswana and Namibia all the way down to South Africa.

TEACHINGS FROM TIME IMMEMORIAL

Kalahari melon is one of the staples in the diet of the San people, magnificent hunter-gatherers who were the first inhabitants of Southern Africa. In 1849, while traveling through the region, explorer David Livingstone documented the cultivation of Cucurbitaceae. The water contained in the *tsamma melo* enabled locals to survive in the desert for weeks at a time, while its seeds, roasted under hot cinders and sometimes ground to a paste, were enjoyed for their high protein content. Crushed and moistened with saliva, they were spread and rubbed on the body to nourish the skin and give it a protective reddish tint.

ON COLLECTING KALAHARI MELON OIL

Harvesting the melons and turning their seeds into oil is traditionally a woman's job. Kalahari melon seed oil is extracted through cold-pressing. It is clear and light, and exudes a nutty aroma.

THE BENEFITS

Kalahari melon seed oil is made up of more than 50% linoleic acid (omega-6), which minimizes the skin's water loss while nourishing and softening it. Oleic acid (omega-9) reinforces the naturally present and protective acid mantle. Palmitic acid is a natural emollient and cleansing component of the cutaneous barrier and the epidermis.

A FEW DROPS

Kalahari melon seed oil works wonders on oily and combination skin. Two or three drops, massaged each night directly onto the face after a gentle yet meticulous cleansing, will be absorbed immediately. In the morning, apply some floral water to facilitate waking up, and there you are—ready for a new day, armed with an even, smooth complexion.

KALAHARI MELON–BASED RECIPES
from Officine Universelle

BALANCE-RESTORING FACIAL FLUID

Your skin has stayed young and is refusing to take sides, switching from dried-out to shiny with no warning. Regular use of this treatment will make it fall in line.

In a small two-ounce jar with a dropper, mix one part Kalahari melon seed oil and one part jojoba oil with ten drops of grapefruit essential oil. Apply a few drops of this detoxifying mixture every night after thorough facial cleansing.

EXTRA-PURIFYING SCRUB

Stimulate your cells with this exfoliating treatment, without overdoing it! Weekly use will suffice to leave your skin silky-smooth.

In a small bowl, mix two tablespoons of Kalahari melon seed oil and one tablespoon of lavender powder with two tablespoons of geranium hydrolate. Use this mixture to gently scrub your face, your neckline area, and even your back, if a soul mate is lending you a hand. Rinse with warm, clear water and pat dry with an immaculately clean cloth.

"The seed is in the fruit and the fruit is in the seed."

ENGLISH PROVERB

✦ KOHL ✦

Powder — Origin: Morocco

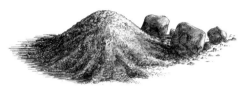

Antimonite

helps prevent and relieve eye infections and protects the eyes from excessive light. In 1565, Mattioli, an Italian physician and botanist, specified that "Antimonite possesses an astringent power and modifies eye ulcers."

PHARAOH'S EYE

With a color that ranges from green to deep black to iridescent midnight blue, antimonite powder is a mineral substance extracted from mountainous rocks in Morocco and Pakistan. Extremely fine, it is said to protect the eyes from infection. This powder known as kohl has a deep, metallic radiance; it is used as an eyeliner throughout the Arabian Peninsula, in the Middle East, in North Africa, and among the peoples of the Sahara, down to the Sudan.

TEACHINGS FROM TIME IMMEMORIAL

In ancient Egypt, kohl was known as *mesdemet*, and its use is documented all the way back to the earliest dynasties of the Old Kingdom. Kohl is reputed to attract the protection of the god Horus by representing the magical Wedjat (or Eye of Horus), contoured with a thick black line. This liner, used to emphasize the eyes, is also valued for its medicinal properties: it

ON COLLECTING KOHL

Kohl recipes are plentiful: each region has — and jealousy protects — its own. It is said that the purest ones come from Sudan, Yemen, and Syria. Chunks of antimonite are first heated to a high temperature to make them highly brittle. Crushed with a mortar and pestle, the resulting antimonite powder is then doused (with rose water . . .) and left to dry, then crushed a second time before finally being sieved. Other ingredients are then commonly added: copper sulfate, carbonized alum, copper carbonate, olive oil, clove powder, musk, pulverized date pits, coral or pearl dust, or even so-called "bat black"!

THE BENEFITS

Galena, or lead sulfide, gives kohl its black, shiny appearance. Phosgenite and laurionite both have bactericidal properties, which explain why it is used to treat conjunctivitis.

A PINCH OF KOHL

Kohl should be applied at night just before bed. It stays on very well, and the more it's used, the more it diffuses its intense presence around the eye that it "chars," creating a natural "smoky eye." Packaged in a small glass vial, it is applied with a small polished wooden stick known as a *mirwed*. The stick is run three times around the inside of the vial; the excess powder is then shaken off with gentle tapping. The stick is placed at the corner of the eye, between the eyelids, and the eyes are then shut. The *mirwed* is then gently swept along the eyelid, and the powder left behind harmoniously accentuates the shape of the eye. The more frequently kohl is used, the more the eye is defined and enhanced.

KOHL-BASED RECIPES
from Officine Universelle

INTENSE KOHL

Kohl recipes are often mysterious. This is a simple version for those who enjoy creating their own makeup.

Place one tablespoon of anthracite kohl and five pinches of midnight blue kohl in a sturdy marble mortar. Add three grains of Melegueta pepper and five pinches of dried jasmine flowers. Crush to a fine powder and sieve several times over. Finish by running the mixture through a very fine-mesh sieve or double layer of cheesecloth, and fill a small glass vial with this preparation, which should be kept in a dry place.

"I have put kohl on my eyelids so that he who looks at me desires me."

EGYPTIAN WISDOM

⬧ KUKUI ⬧

Nut, oil — Origin: Pacific Islands

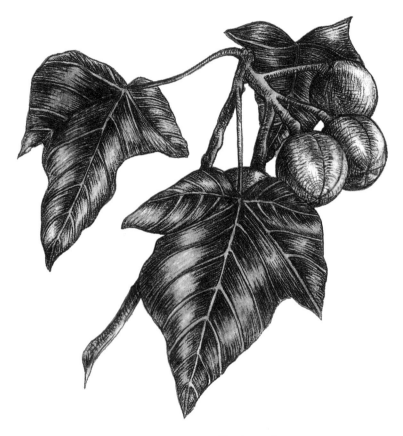

Aleurites moluccana

THE WALNUT
OF THE TROPICS

This evergreen tree, with its majestic wide bearing, thrives in the tropics, offering up the desirable shade of its pretty palmate leaves, which are home to numerous species of birds. Following a spectacular white inflorescence, *Aleurites moluccana* adorns itself with nuts. The candlenut tree grows throughout the Pacific region under a number of different names: *ama* in the Marquesas Islands, *lama* in Samoa, and *ti'a'iri* in Tahiti.

> *"A kukui provides as much shelter as a house."*

tree of Hawai'i. *Lei kukui*, i.e., necklaces made from kukui nuts, were the preferred adornment of local chiefs; nowadays they are still worn by dancers during rituals honoring Lono, the god of agriculture. Canoes and surfboards used to be carved from its trunk, and its oil was rubbed on to caulk them and make them waterproof.

TEACHINGS FROM TIME IMMEMORIAL

The handsome kukui is a providential tree for all Pacific Islanders, and seems possessed of limitless talents. Its oil is said to heal minor skin complaints and have purgative properties. A fresh leaf, perched atop one's head, was said by the ancients to soothe headaches. Simply chewed, the seeds have a cleansing effect. The soot left over after burning the nuts and kernels makes a fine tattoo ink: a small serrated comb made of bone, tortoiseshell, or nacre and fixed to a short wooden handle is dipped in soot mixed with monoï, and repeated pricks on the skin cause micro-incisions that allow the pigment to be deposited inside the epidermis. Kukui kernels are also used to make hourglass candles: they are strung on a vegetable stem and burn one after the other. . . . In 1816, in his new dictionary of natural history, Jacques Eustache de Sève cited the candlenut tree and its uses: "The latter is cultivated for its nut, whose oil is widely traded." In 1862, in a book about the resources of the island of Réunion, G. Imhaus asserted that "the leaves of this tree are potent sudorifics." An oil factory has been in existence in Tahiti since the 19th century. In 1959, it became the official

ON COLLECTING KUKUI NUTS

Kukui nuts are harvested once they have fallen from the tree. Extracting the oil is hard work: heating the nuts to 203°F and plunging them in a bath of cold water is necessary to break their shell. The kernels are cold-pressed and the oil is purified mechanically. This delicate oil, with its yellow tint, low viscosity, and very "dry" feel, absorbs very easily. It can quickly oxidize and must be kept refrigerated for no more than six months.

THE BENEFITS

Kukui nut oil is rich in linoleic acid (omega-6 and omega-3), which protects the skin from external aggressions and efficiently prevents it from drying out. Its high oleic acid content (omega-9) nourishes the skin, helps with scarification, reduces minor lesions, and soothes itching.

A FEW DROPS

Soothing and nourishing kukui oil is the perfect oil for those who do not like . . . oils! Indeed, its dry, nongreasy feel is a blessing for anyone who does not relish the customary feel of oils on their skin. Its consummate dryness enables it to take good care of sensitive, irritated skin. It is ideal for children. A dash of kukui oil and lavender hydrolate splashed onto a cotton pad makes the best possible facial cleanser for so-called problem-prone skin. After shampooing, a few drops in the hollow of your palm will condition the curls and lengths of dry hair. Beware, though: kukui oil is fragile and must be used quickly.

KUKUI-BASED RECIPES
from Officine Universelle

GREAT PACIFIC
FACIAL CLEANSE

Once a month, perform this great tropical cleanse: a surefire balance-restoring radiance booster—and what's left of the fruit will surely be eaten!

In a bowl, using a fork, crush a tablespoon of papaya flesh and pour a scant teaspoon of kukui oil on top. Gently rub this mixture on the face, avoiding the area around the eyes, then leave on for five minutes. Remove this mask using a tissue, without rubbing the skin, and rinse with warm water.

ISLAND
HAIR MASK

Instead of patronizing the boring haircare aisles, prepare your own nourishing mask just as you would a culinary dish!

Mix a very ripe banana and add 2½ teaspoons of kukui oil. Add half a puréed avocado and five teaspoons of coconut milk. Whisk this mixture together until you get a rich, smooth mask. Apply immediately to unwashed, dry hair. Leave on for about fifteen minutes, then remove the excess with a comb. Finally, wash the hair with a gentle shampoo, then rinse with cold water mixed with a tablespoon of cider vinegar.

⸙ LAVENDER ⸙

Powder, hydrolate, and essential oil (flowers) — Origin: Persia

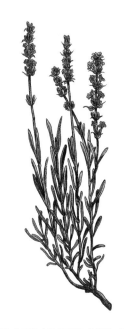

Lavandula

THE STRAIGHT AND NARROW

L avender's violet and pungently aromatic stalk delights the eye and the other senses. The plant numbers three main varieties: true lavender (also known as "narrow-leaved lavender"), broadleaved lavender, and hybrid lavender—a cross of the other two. Hybrid lavender is six times more productive than its progenitors; it is best suited for the preparation of the lavender sachets that perfume the inside of wardrobes, or for minor cosmetic uses, while true lavender remains the variety that is most highly prized by high perfumery and has been included in the formulation of remedies and treatment recipes since antiquity.

TEACHINGS FROM TIME IMMEMORIAL

In the Middle Ages, the plant gained its current name, derived from the Latin *lavare*: Romans used to throw it in their bathwater to perfume and purify it. The fair washerwomen of way back when used to add twigs of lavender to their detergent to harness the same virtues. Following the plagues and other epidemics that coursed through the Provence region from the 5th to the 18th centuries, lavender's medicinal properties were studied and put to use. It was reputed to ward off and destroy lethal miasmas, and was notably included in the composition of "Four Thieves Vinegar": those who were in contact with the diseased and plague-stricken used to anoint themselves with this concoction to avoid contagion. Along with camphor crystals, lavender was included in the "fainting pads" that ladies used to sniff when gripped by some sudden rush of emotion. In India, Ayurvedic medicine recommends it to cure depression. As early as the 17th century, the chemists of the Lure mountain, a range in Haute Provence that was famed for the exceptional quality of its true lavender and for its cultivation of other "simple" herbs, made brisk trade of it. In the 18th century, Giovanni Maria Farina, the famed Italian perfumer, met with success throughout Europe thanks to his "Aqua Mirabilis," formulated with (among other ingredients) true lavender.

The plant's renown increased in the 19th century; Provençal peasants invested in mobile alembics, the better to perform distillation themselves between harvests. The town of Grasse became the most highly reputed production center of lavender essence.

Until it became so common that it now perfumes even the lowliest household cleaning products (made with hybrid lavender, of course . . .), the magical scent of lavender used to be deemed precious, intense, complex, and unique. Casanova perfumed his stationery with the plant and burned its dry stems inside his house to foster harmony and peace.

ON COLLECTING LAVENDER

From April to September, the flower is a source of delight for bees and other pollinating insects, striating the Provence countryside with its purple-blue streaks. The best lavender fields are to be found on plateaus located at altitudes of 1,970 to 4,595 feet. The plant's calyxed flowers, whose essential oil has a wild and pungent scent, are harvested when the petals begin to wilt. The flowering tops are left to dry, mixed, and hand-picked so as to remove all impurities. Lavender flowers are then distilled to produce what perfumers call an "extract" and aromatherapists call an "essential oil." They yield a potent floral water and can also be crushed to a powder.

THE BENEFITS

Lavender is beneficial to the nervous system: it helps fight insomnia, headaches, and irritability, and alleviates depression. Monoterpenols and monoterpenes harmonize, calm, and soothe. The esters it contains are famously antispasmodic, anti-inflammatory, and sedative. It is also recommended for the treatment of wounds and burns, as well as eczema. Finally, lavender is an excellent antiparasitic.

A FEW DROPS
AND A FEW TWIGS

It's bedtime! Two drops of *Lavandula angustifolia* on the flat fringes of a pillowcase are an invitation to sleep the sleep of the just. Alternatively, massage your temples with fresh lavender flowers before bed to ensure sweet dreams. Spraying a few measures of lavender floral water on a sunburn will soothe its fiery discomfort. A few lavender twigs will suffice to perfume a wardrobe or a drawer and infuse it with the memory of summer—what's more, mites do not relish the plant's fragrance as much as we do.

LAVENDER-BASED RECIPES

from Officine Universelle

❈

"MOOD-ALTERING" LAVENDER BATH

Are you feeling down and irritable? Dip into a milky lavender bath and head for the bed once your spirit has been soothed! You'll finally forget about everything in Morpheus's embrace.

In a coffee grinder, crush three tablespoons of dried lavender flowers to a powder, then add two tablespoons of organic whole milk and two tablespoons of (heated) organic milk. Whisk together and pour into a hot bath.

Step into this bath (after showering, obviously), breathe deeply, and relax.

PURIFYING FACIAL STEAM BATH

This highly effective purifying steam bath, followed by a clay mask, is conducive to clear skin and fresh ideas.

Bring to a boil two cups of mineral water with two tablespoons of fresh lavender flowers (or dried flowers if you don't have any fresh) and two tablespoons of rosemary leaves and flowers. Cover and allow to infuse for ten minutes. Place your face over the scented water, under a clean dry cloth. Enjoy this steam bath for five minutes. It is most potent to calm and improve oily and combination skin.

DREAM NIGHT PILLOW

Feathers are so banal . . . bring the leaf-and-flower pillow back into fashion! For the perfect nap, a long plane trip, or as a companion for your most restful nights.

Pad a large rectangle of cotton with a fragrant and soothing mix of flowers and leaves—then fold it and sew it shut. It is recommended to choose a finely woven cloth to ensure the leaves do not pierce through, or to cover the pillow with a second case. The mixture inside should comprise 2.65 ounces of the following dried plants: lavender and chamomile flowers, holy basil, California poppy, and lemon balm leaves. Adjust this composition depending on your olfactory preferences.

"Washerwoman, washerwoman! Have you seen the blue fish That was swimming in the river? He was bringing you lavender, lavender in a blue bunch."

R. DESNOS

⟡ LEMON ⟡

Fruit, bark, and essential oil — Origin: Far East

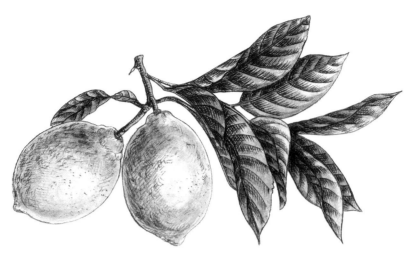

Citrus limon

THE FRUIT OF
THE MEDIAN KINGDOM

◦

Citrus fruits make up a large family that originates from the Far East and later reached the West via the passage of time and civilization. The citron probably came first. The modern lemon tree is reportedly a hybrid of the lime, the grapefruit, and this original citron, *Citrus medica*, the "Median apple," as Virgil calls it in the *Georgics*. The Arabs brought the lemon along with them during their expansion around the Mediterranean; nowadays it is cultivated along its shores. The numerous varieties of this citrus fruit are distinguished by their shape; the thickness and color of their rind; the number, size, and tint of their pips; and of course their taste and scent.

TEACHINGS FROM TIME
IMMEMORIAL

◦

Called *limûn* in Persian, it became *limone* in Italian. From Alexander the Great to the Arab conquerors, from the Crusaders to Christopher Columbus, explorers, sailors, and adventurers have contributed to its worldwide dissemination — most likely because it protected sailors from dreadful scurvy, which used to decimate ship crews. Richer in vitamin C than its cousin the orange, and generous in bioflavonoids, the lemon protects blood capillaries. At the turn of the first millennium, the famed Persian physician Avicenna recommended it for palpitations. Lemon juice also has a reputation as an antidote against the effects of poisons and venoms. The pips were formerly used as a vermifuge and a medicine to fight fevers. The Chinese mentioned it in the 12th century. Acclimatized in the West by Crusaders upon their return from the Middle East, the lemon began to be cultivated everywhere as a "simple" fruit, and entered into the Western pharmacopeia. It thrives in Southern France, especially on what we now call the French Riviera. Menton has been producing lemon essence since the 11th century, and has been exporting it since the Renaissance. By the 19th century, the lemon's reputation was firmly established; Paul Lacroix, aka Jacob the Bibliophile, recommended its cosmetic use: "The acidic juice of oranges, lemons, etc., cleanses the skin very well, removes the grime that clings to its surface, and is beneficial when mixed with bathwater." It is reputed to brighten the complexion, to attenuate dimples and to purify. In India, a lemon hung above a door is considered a protective good-luck charm.

ON PREPARING LEMONS

Lemons are harvested between April and July. Their outside envelope—the pericarp—is lightly to heavily bumpy and shot through with tiny pouches, filled with an aromatic liquid that contains the fruit's essence. Under the outer skin is a white, spongy pith called the albedo. Then comes the pulp of the fruit, divided into segments. For the cold extraction of lemon essential oil, the fruit is both pressed and grated. A centrifuge separates the essential oil from the resulting juice. It is also possible to grate the rind the old-fashioned way, to physically rupture the aromatic pouches.

THE BENEFITS

Lemon bestows its benefits with great largesse: vitamin C stimulates the epidermis, activates blood and lymphatic microcirculation, and helps with scarification by promoting synthesis of collagen and elastin. It also reduces the thickness of the *stratum corneum*. Magnesium and calcium support the proper functioning of the skin's enzymatic systems. Bioflavonoids work to protect the cells from the oxidation caused by free radicals. Pectin and limonene have well-known antiseptic and anti-inflammatory properties. Citric acid is an ideal bactericide and fungicide.

A LITTLE ZEST

Lemon will play along with all of your cosmetic preparations. It is included in numerous masks, bath products and serums. In its simplest garb, it will perfectly cleanse the most damaged, stained hands—after gardening for instance. Follow in the footsteps of Lola Montez, who shared a lemon-based hand beauty recipe in her work *The Arts of Beauty* (1858). Half a pure lemon simply rubbed on the nails and hands will leave the skin clean and the nails smooth and properly white. It also makes for an ideal natural deodorant: rubbing the armpits with some fresh lemon leftovers will put a stop to the proliferation of undesirable bacteria. Beware in the sunshine, though: lemon contains photosensitizing molecules.

LEMON-BASED RECIPES

from Officine Universelle

SHINE WATER

Bring radiance to your blond or light brown hair by taking the time to rinse it with a simple lemon-based water.

Dilute the juice of a lemon in a bottle of mineral water and rinse your hair with this water after shampooing.

SOFTEST BODY WRAP

This wrap should be performed in the springtime, so that the body is ready to appear in full light again. . . .

Prepare a large towel on a bed or a bench. After bathing or showering, on dried skin, apply a wrap made from the following ingredients: the juice of one lemon, five tablespoons of honey, and two tablespoons of plum kernel oil. Leave on for fifteen minutes, resting comfortably on the towel, then rinse with warm water.

QUEENLY FEET

To parade around in your sandals, Lola Montez–style, it's best to tread lightly.

In a small tub of water filled to a third of its capacity, pour the freshly pressed juice of one whole lemon, half a glass of sake, and three tablespoons of colorless eau-de-vie. Bathe your feet for five minutes and scrub the nails with a small, soft brush. Towel dry with a spotlessly clean cloth, without forgetting the spaces between your toes.

SUGAR-LEMON WAXING PASTE

Hair and beauty canons are old foes. The fight is a painful and ruthless one: the Eastern version requires a certain amount of dexterity, but efficiently gets rid of unsightly hairiness and exfoliates the legs magnificently.

In a heavy-bottomed saucepan, pour the filtered juice of two lemons onto six sugar cubes with a tablespoon of water. Melt the sugar and stir with a wooden spoon until you get an amber-colored paste. Pour on an oiled slab of marble, work the paste until soft with fingers dipped in cold water, and shape it into a ball. With a firm hand, spread over a small patch of clean, not-yet-moisturized skin, then yank the paste right off, taking the hairs along with it.

"A bitter truth is better than a sweet lie."

RUSSIAN WISDOM

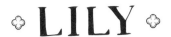

✦ LILY ✦

Macerate (petals, bulb) — Origin: Asia Minor

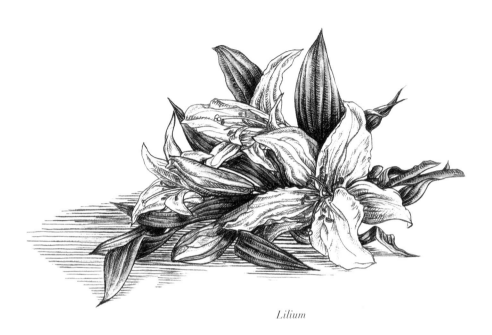

Lilium

"I AM THE ROSE OF SHARON, AND THE LILY OF THE VALLEYS"

◉

In the wild, *Lilium* is a plant that numbers more than a hundred varieties, grouped in two families: one from Asia and the other more specifically from East Asia. The flower can be differentiated by its appearance and its pungent aroma. A symbol of innocence and purity, the lily has been known as the Virgin Mary's flower since the Middle Ages. This "Madonna Lily," *Lilium candidum*, with its large inflorescence of ample white corollas, is used for its cosmetic benefits.

TEACHINGS FROM TIME IMMEMORIAL

◉

According to the ancient Greeks, this "flower of flowers" was born of a drop of the goddess Hera's milk, which fell to the ground as she was breastfeeding Heracles. Since the dawn of time and the world over, the lily has been a symbol of beauty, majesty, maternity, and purity. The Romans used white lily petals to soothe burns. Left to macerate in oil or alcohol, these petals were reputed to alleviate skin conditions such as rosacea, as well as the onset of freckles—vagaries of melanin that ran afoul of beauty ideals that favored alabaster complexions. . . . Jean-Louis Fargeon, Marie-Antoinette's famed perfumer, praised its brightening properties: "The fragrant water that can be extracted from lily flowers, using the heat of a bain-marie, is the preferred means of improving maidens' complexions; it removes marks from their faces, especially when mixed with a little salt of tartar."

"Wise is the man who, having two loaves of bread, sells one to buy a lily."

CHINESE PROVERB

ON COLLECTING AND PREPARING THE MACERATE

Fresh lily flowers are left to macerate in a neutral vegetable oil, such as sunflower. The resulting macerate has a very pale yellow tint, and its scent is very light. In order to concoct your macerate, cut the (untreated) open flowers in the early morning, remove the pistils, and gently wipe each petal before proceeding with the preparation, as per our recipe on page 136.

THE BENEFITS

The phytosterols that are naturally present in lily petals have potent anti-inflammatory and antioxidant properties. They soothe and improve skin quality. Linoleic acid (omega-6) fights drying and helps achieve proper hydration. Etiolin treats pigmentation issues and efficiently helps even out and brighten skin tone.

A FEW DROPS

White lily macerate is an ally of skin that is prone to staining or to bearing the marks of sun exposure. For after-sun care, it can be mixed with an equal amount of sesame oil. To care for the neckline area, white lily macerate and daisy macerate make a happy match. And as far as the hands are concerned, combining the macerate with a drop of castor seed oil is ideal to make them look radiant and youthful again.

LILY-BASED RECIPES

from Officine Universelle

WHITE LILY
YOUTH ELIXIR

Ancestral beauty treatments were formulated using the treasures of both the garden and the wilderness. Vacations are the best time to reconnect with these habits by preparing your first macerate.

Place three handfuls of white lily petals (with the stamens and pistils removed and gently wiped) in a freshly sterilized jar. You may complement this maceration with a bunch of parsley to boost the complexion's radiance, a handful of daisies for a more firming effect, or a handful of marigold flowers for an even more effective action against brown spots. Pour three tablespoons plus one teaspoon of grapeseed oil over the petals and seal the jar hermetically, making sure the petals remain immersed. Allow to macerate for three weeks, making sure the jar is exposed to the sun's rays every morning. Filter and store in one or several small jars with droppers. This oil is a natural treatment that is highly efficient in preventing skin aging.

AT SUMMER'S END,
A LILY COMPLEXION

Steam baths are some of the simplest and most beneficial facial treatments. A few minutes are enough to brighten the complexion and relax the mind.

Drop a few white lily petals in a fine-mesh sieve over some simmering mineral water. Cover with a lid, remove from the heat, and wait for a few minutes. As soon as the heat becomes reasonably bearable, expose your face to this luxurious steam bath for a few minutes.

⟡ LOOFAH ⟡

Vegetable land sponge — Origin: India

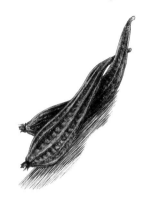

Luffa acutangula, Luffa aegyptiaca, and Luffa cylindrica

SCRATCH ME IF YOU CAN

◦

This fibrous climbing plant from the Cucurbitaceae family has tropical origins and used to thrive in India. Nowadays, it is cultivated from Southeast Asia to Africa. Its sturdy, downy, and angular stems bear fruits that are barely edible when they reach full maturity after four months—although in Asia they are sometimes harvested for cooking when still young and small.

TEACHINGS FROM TIME IMMEMORIAL

◦

The loofah's botanical name derives from the Egyptian Arabic word *luff*, and its moniker varies from one country and one language to the next: *ansangokan* in Benin, *napé* in Senegal, *nabébé* in Mali. Once prepared and dried, this type of gourd reveals a dense, fibrous structure, which resembles a sponge or sometimes a rag. Its fresh leaves were also once used to treat skin infections.

ON COLLECTING LOOFAH

◦

The fruit must be harvested at full maturity, when its skin starts turning brown. Peeled, it then reveals a whole network of white fibers. This fibrous slab is immersed in water for several days, then shaken vigorously to be rid of its pulp and seeds entirely. Finally, it is blanched in boiling water. The most esteemed loofah comes from Egypt: its suppleness and its ability to absorb are much lauded.

THE BENEFITS

◦

This exfoliating sponge can absorb up to twenty times its weight in water and has the most natural scrubbing effect on the body. It stimulates the skin through friction when exfoliating and encourages lymphatic drainage.

JUST ONE PIECE

A piece of loofah can be run over the whole body, except for the face. When wet, it rids the body of surface impurities and dead skin cells. It can be used once or twice a week, especially towards the end of winter to renew the skin, or in summer to care for a suntan. After use, the loofah must be rinsed very carefully with clear water and left out to dry.

⟡ LOTUS ⟡

Powder (seeds) — Origin: India

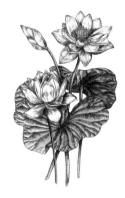

Nelumbo nucifera

THE SACRED FLOWER

◉

This rare and fascinating species has but two varieties: the Indian lotus and the American lotus. This aquatic plant grows wild in the warm regions of Asia. Its large leaves are host to magnificent, fragrantly scented, solitary flowers that float on the calm and marshy waters where this rhizomic plant thrives. During periods of pollination, these flowers play a thermotactic role, maintaining the plant at its ideal temperature, 86°F — a reasonable level of heat that is favorable to its development. Engineers are enthralled by the hydrophobic and self-cleansing properties of lotus leaves.

TEACHINGS FROM TIME IMMEMORIAL

◉

The lotus is the national flower of both India and Vietnam; it is considered sacred in Buddhism, and is ubiquitous in Asian arts and traditions as a symbol of life, rebirth, and longevity. The flower emerges radiant and pure out of murky waters, embodying the aspiration to purity held by all living things. The Buddha is often depicted on a lotus, in expectation of enlightenment or nirvana, in the so-called "lotus" position — sitting cross-legged with a straight back, each foot resting on the opposite thigh. On the banks and delta of the Nile, the plant was valued as far back as antiquity for its medicinal properties and its subtle fragrance.

Everything in this noble flower is useful and precious: the seeds can be enjoyed boiled or roasted; the young leaves are eaten cooked and fried; the rhizome is crushed to produce a prized flour; and the stamens make excellent infusions and are included in perfume recipes. Chinese medicine prescribes the flower to cure fevers as well as liver ailments. Ayurveda recommends eating the seeds and roots to increase the body's tonus and stimulate blood flow; the flower is also praised as an aphrodisiac.

ON COLLECTING LOTUS SEEDS

◉

Protected by their envelope, lotus seeds boast an exceptional longevity and keep easily. This certainly accounts for the view of the flower as a symbol of rebirth. They are harvested by hand, dried, and crushed to a powder.

THE BENEFITS

The flavonoids that occur naturally in the lotus's seeds stimulate microcirculation and fortify blood vessels. Saponin is an antiseptic as well as an efficient cleansing agent that is gentle on the skin. High concentrations of phenols, which are antioxidants, have a stimulating and toning action. The plant is reportedly able to fight the effects of aging by warding off free radicals.

"The soul unfolds, much like a lotus with countless petals."

KHALIL GIBRAN

A FEW PINCHES

Lotus powder is included in the formulation of energizing facial treatments. This use restores the complexion's radiance and overall quality. One gram of lotus powder may be added to a small vial of facial oil to enhance it with the seed's properties. Nothing can ensure facial relaxation quite like lotus powder!

LOTUS-BASED RECIPES
from Officine Universelle

SACRED LOTUS ENLIGHTENING MASK

The serenity and radiance of the lotus flower can be yours: enhance your clay-based mask with this rare powder.

Mix one teaspoon of lotus powder with two teaspoons of white clay, one tablespoon of orange blossom hydrolate, and three drops of lemon essential oil. Apply this mask to the face and neck. Sit in the lotus position, breathe deeply, and reach a state of quiet for fifteen minutes. Rinse with warm water and pat dry with a clean cloth.

⟡ MARIGOLD ⟡

Flowers, macerate — Origin: Mediterranean region

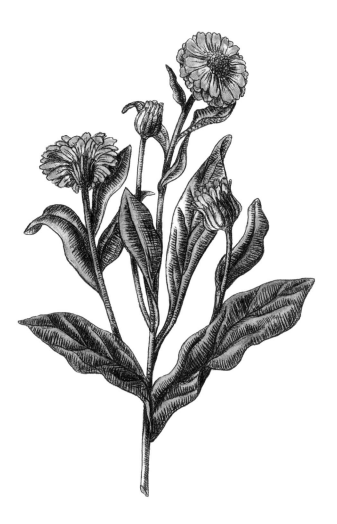

Calendula officinalis

IN THE SUN

❦

The officinal "pot" marigold and the "field" marigold are held in equal esteem. Their uses and compositions are interrelated and rather similar. Originating from Southern Europe, the plant and its radiant orange-yellow flower are perfectly happy in all temperate regions. Acting as the gardener's valuable auxiliary, the marigold naturally wards off aphids and is cultivated in kitchen gardens to protect the crops from pests.

"Some painters turn the sun into a yellow dot; others turn a yellow dot into the sun."

PABLO PICASSO

TEACHINGS FROM TIME IMMEMORIAL

Named after the Latin *calendae*, "the first days of the month," the marigold's flower is, as the Dominican friar Albert le Grand beautifully put it, "the bride of the sun," whose radiance it seems to borrow. This idea inspired one of its French names, *solsequier*: "that which follows the sun." The more trivial English name, pot marigold, evokes its tinctorial use in the kitchen, to perfume and dye soups. It was also used to revive the plumage of canaries! This great classic of Western phytotherapy has been cultivated throughout Europe since the 9th century, as recommended by Charlemagne in his ordinance *De villis vel curtis imperii*. In the late 19th century, the abbot Sebastian Kneipp prescribed it to alleviate varicose veins and skin conditions. In homeopathy, it has remained the undisputed panacea in caring for small, minor wounds.

ON COLLECTING MARIGOLD

Marigold flowers must be harvested in the morning. Soaked in dew, the flowers are then put out to dry. The flowering tops are left to macerate for a month, immersed in a neutral virgin oil, thus gradually yielding their properties. The fragrance of marigold macerate is strong, but not cloying.

THE BENEFITS

Marigold macerate, often called calendula macerate, is softening, antiseptic, and healing: in fact the flower's petals have a high concentration of flavonoids, triterpene-diols, and saponines, which are all effective against inflammation and irritation.

A FEW PETALS

Marigold macerate is a bathroom essential for the whole family: applied topically as an ointment, it soothes baby skin flare-ups, razor burn, and small blemishes. Remember that in the olden days, bathing in water infused with fresh or dried marigold flowers was said to attract the respect and admiration of whoever you met during the day. Keep that in mind on the eve of an important meeting or rendezvous! And of course, if you find yourself deep in the wild, away from any chemical treatment, eat marigold flowers: they have a fresh and crisp radish-like flavor.

MARIGOLD-BASED RECIPES

from Officine Universelle

THE GREAT BLOND RINSING WATER

Blond hair, you say? Here is a chance to play with light, and hairstyles—braids even—as a nod to some of our ancestors, the Vikings. . . .

Prepare a decoction of two fistfuls of dried marigold flowers in two cups of mineral water. Once it has cooled down, filter it, pour it into a bottle, and add a tablespoon of cider vinegar. Of course, you should not rinse your hair after use. Keep refrigerated and use within a week.

THE THOUSAND-VIRTUE OINTMENT

Make the most of a summer in the countryside by creating your own marigold-based ointment for pesky skin troubles.

In a sterilized glass jar with a wide opening, allow one ounce of calendula petals to macerate in ¾ cup of sunflower oil for three weeks. This maceration is best left to rest on a windowsill, where it will catch the sun's rays. The flowers must always be immersed in the oil. Shake lightly every day. Filter through cheesecloth.

In a bain-marie over low heat, melt one ounce of beeswax in the macerate. Fill a sterilized glass jar with this preparation and allow it to set. Keep away from direct sunlight and use within three months. Use it to care for any itch, redness, or irritation.

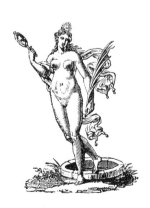

❖ MARULA ❖

Kernels, oil — Origin: South Africa

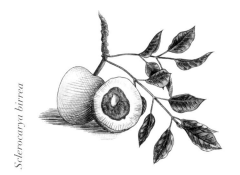

Sclerocarya birrea

THE KING OF TREES

○

The growth of the marula on the African continent followed the migratory movements of the Bantu peoples, who consider it a tree of life. This African plum tree stretches its branches heavenward in the savanna and *bushveld*. In the warmer months it's covered in yellow fruit, which the elephants have a craving for. The fruit quickly ferments in their stomach, making the pachyderms "drunk!"

TEACHINGS FROM TIME IMMEMORIAL

○

In Zimbabwe, on the archaeological site of Pomongwe Cave, which dates back to the Middle Stone Age, marula fruits were already being consumed in abundance. A true treasure of African botany, the generous female tree is one of the continent's most fructiferous. The fruit is eaten raw, cooked into a jelly, or fermented to make beer and other types

of alcohol. Its therapeutic and practical properties are numerous: its bark, after decoction, is reputed to heal dysentery and to calm malarial symptoms; the gum that is extracted from its branches makes for a strong ink; the infusion of its fruit yields a potent natural insecticide.

ON COLLECTING MARULA OIL

○

Once picked, peeled, and dried in the sun, the fruit's hardy stones are crushed in order to free the kernels they protect. These kernels are very rich and just as generous: after pressing, they yield an oil that is oxidation-resistant and therefore more stable, meaning that it keeps better than other oils. In Namibia, it is customarily women who produce marula oil, which they use both to hydrate their skin and to help preserve meats.

THE BENEFITS

○

The vitamin C content of a marula fruit is four times as high as that of an orange. This elevated concentration stimulates cell turnover and cutaneous microcirculation. The presence of vitamin E helps protect cells from oxidation. Oleic acid (omega-9) and palmitic acid maintain the skin's elasticity and hydration.

A FEW DROPS

Regular application of marula oil to the face, after freshening up with some geranium hydrolate, will valiantly shield you from irritation and the whips and scorns of time. The oil evens out the epidermis and tightens the grain, leaving the skin smooth and firm. Experience has shown that while marula oil is suited to all skin types, it is particularly beneficial to combination skin.

MARULA-BASED RECIPES

from Officine Universelle

FACIAL BALANCING TREATMENT

Time passes, but some of the frustrations of adolescent skin continue to manifest themselves in stressful times. Breathe deeply and sleep soundly with the nightly application of this efficient treatment to freshly cleansed skin.

In a small two-ounce jar with a dropper, mix one part marula oil and one part nigella oil with three drops of tea tree essential oil and one drop of clove essential oil.

SUNNY DAY BODY TREATMENT

With the arrival of summer comes the joy of reuniting with your bathing suit! Stay calm— getting ready for it can be fun. Follow a daily vigorous brushing with application of this hair-growth-slowing, anti-cellulite treatment.

In a three-ounce jar with a dropper, mix one part marula oil and one part nut grass oil, enhancing this combination with ten drops of Atlas cedar essential oil and one or two drops of, for example, patchouli essential oil, to get that comforting scent.

"The heart is like a tree, it grows where it wishes."

AFRICAN PROVERB

✦ MINT ✦

Essential oil, hydrolate (leaves) — Origin: Great Britain

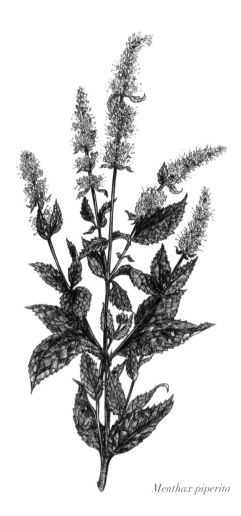

Menthax piperita

TINGLING PLANT

T his delicious, pungently aromatic plant from the odoriferous Lamiaceae family grows readily throughout Europe, the Mediterranean, Western Asia, and Northern Africa. Its deep green leaves exude an intoxicating scent at dusk, spreading their fragrance at the merest touch. Mint thrives and gains ground wherever it is acclimatized, thanks to its invasive underground stolons. These botanic "scouts" radiate all around the root, enabling easy crossing between different varieties. Peppermint is thus the happy and tasty marriage of Asian mint and spearmint!

TEACHINGS FROM TIME IMMEMORIAL

❦

Ancient myths have it that the nymph Minthe, so beautiful and so pale, was coveted by the blacksmith god, the infernal Hades. This infatuation angered his wife, Persephone, and his mother-in-law, Demeter. Together, they transformed young Minthe into a wild plant—mint. Could this amorous origin have paved the way for its reputation as an aphrodisiac? Roman naturalist Pliny the Elder considered mint to be efficacious in several respects. In his *Natural History*, he listed its properties and medicinal uses at length. Purifying and purgative, it was reputed to combat numerous afflictions, from the simplest to the most complex. He already noted that a few sprigs would efficiently purify water and prevent milk from going sour. Roman women used to chew a paste of mint and honey to freshen their breath. Although mint always ornamented the monk-tended gardens of "simples," peppermint did not officially enter the traditional European pharmacopeia until the late 17th century, when the English naturalist John Ray set it apart from other mints. In 1721, it made its entrance into the registry of remedies of the city of London, and has since become one of the most widely used medicinal herbs.

ON COLLECTING

❦

The harvest of mint leaves occurs in June and July, just before blooming: their essential oil content is then at its peak. The floral water and the essential oil are obtained by distillation of the fresh leaves. Eight hundred eighty pounds of mint leaves are then needed to yield one precious quart of essential oil.

ON VIRTUES

❦

The powers of the peppermint leaf are numerous. It concentrates flavonoids, triterpenes, and phenol acids, which help cells fight oxidation and help reduce inflammations. The pro-vitamin A carotenoid pigments it contains soothe irritations, while their tannins have astringent and protective properties. Peppermint essential oil contains menthol and some of its derivatives: its refreshing effect is due to the activation of cold-sensitive chemical captors located under the skin. This early sensation is accompanied by a beneficial decongesting and anti-inflammatory action.

A FEW DROPS

Peppermint essential oil, much like all of its peers, must be consumed wisely and cautiously. It must never be used to care for children or pregnant women. For others, it should always be diluted down to 5% in a vegetable oil for external use: it can then be enjoyed to soothe skin irritations, calm sunburn, or procure a delightfully refreshing sensation.

MINT-BASED RECIPES

from Officine Universelle

BYE BYE BLUES

When in need of a pick-me-up, or a comforting piece of candy, try lifting your spirits by giving them the green treatment. These mint compresses soothe headaches, pacify the mood, and refresh the mien. A touch of lipstick, the benevolent ear of a girlfriend, and you are back!

In a saucepan, bring a large glass of water to a simmer and throw a generous fistful of mint leaves in there. Remove from the heat and allow to infuse for ten minutes. Soak a compress with the mint water and wring it out, then apply it on the face and eyelids. This will chase away headaches and irritations, smooth out your facial features, and perk up your sense of humor.

MENTHOL BODY SCRUB

A warm-day treatment to get ready for summer dresses.

Mix a cup of freshly chopped mint leaves with four tablespoons of coarse salt and four tablespoons of sweet almond oil. Add two or three drops of peppermint essential oil. This mixture will keep for a month in the fridge in an airtight container. Rub this mixture vigorously over all areas of the body that seem to require it. Rinse under the shower or by dipping into a bath.

RELAXING AROMATIC MINT BATH

Experiment with mint and its purifying virtues to improve the quality of the municipal water in your bath.

Pour some mineral water into a large stockpot. Turn up the heat and throw in a handful of wild mint, thyme, and sage, plus a handful of rose petals, before the water reaches a boil. Simmer for a few minutes, remove from the heat, and allow to infuse for five minutes. Skim the water and remove the botanicals. Draw yourself a warm bath, add the infused water, and dip into the bathtub for about twenty minutes. Pat yourself dry with a towel and go lie down under some warm covers for fifteen minutes.

PURIFYING MIST

Why not institute beauty rituals for the whole family? Take advantage of a family vacation to experiment and let your younglings or your special someone benefit from your cosmetic creations.

Bring two cups of mineral water to a boil with two tablespoons of mint leaves and a fine sprig of thyme. Cover and allow to infuse for ten minutes. Place your face over the scented water, under a clean, dry cloth. Enjoy this steam bath for five minutes.

The whole family will find its skin refreshed!

❖ MISWAK ❖

Twigs, bark, and roots — Origin: West Africa

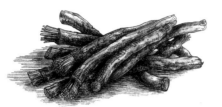

Salvadora persica

TOOTH WOOD

◦

Salvadora persica, a small tree with a crooked trunk and a fragrant bark, called *miswak*, *siwak*, or *arak* depending on the region, thrives in Asia and Africa. Nowadays, it is especially cultivated in Yemen, East Africa, India, and Saudi Arabia.

TEACHINGS FROM TIME IMMEMORIAL

◦

As early as antiquity, miswak use was reputed to treat the teeth, purify the mouth, and perfume the breath. The twigs, bark, and roots can be chewed and constitute a sort of solid toothpaste. Half a century before our era, the Indian surgeon Sushruta already listed sixty-seven dental pathologies in his medical treatise—and prescribed the use of miswak to cure many of them. The hadiths report that "using miswak purifies the mouth and pleases the lord." Today, the World Health Organization strongly recommends it for oro-dental care, and it is one of the most widely used tooth cleansers in Asia and the Middle East.

ON COLLECTING MISWAK

◦

Miswak can be used dried or fresh. When fresh, the tip of the stick is to be chewed and then used as a brush with which to rub the teeth and gums. When dry, the stick must first be dipped in hot water or an infusion of sage, thyme, etc., to soften its fibers and allow the same action to be performed.

THE BENEFITS

◦

Everything is inside miswak: the fluorine it naturally contains wards off cavities and strengthens the enamel. Vitamin C revitalizes the gums and reduces their occasional bleeding due to dental plaque. Saponins have antiseptic, cleansing, and purifying properties. Minerals such as potassium, sodium, and calcium, among others, whiten and strengthen the enamel.

JUST A STICK

During your travels, when faced with the wonderful spread of an Eastern shop, purchase a bit of miswak. Chew, gnaw, bite, and let yourself be surprised by its green, spicy taste. Miswak is also available as a powder: sprinkle a pinch of wood powder on your toothpaste to boost its aroma and enhance its action.

❖ MONGONGO ❖

Oil (nuts) — Origin: Botswana

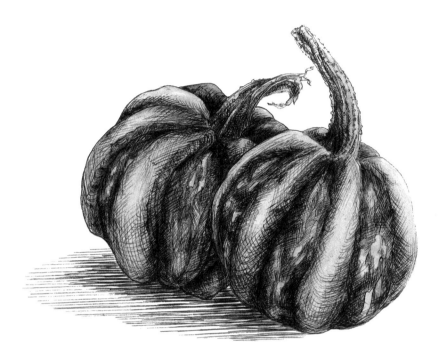

Schinziophyton rautanenii

THE HUNTER'S NUT

❀

This beautiful tree thrives on the hillsides and dunes of the South African savannas and the Kalahari in particular. It is valued for its fruit, which is a staple of the local diet, and for the oil extracted from its nuts. The fair fiber of manketti wood (the mongongo's other name) stands in contrast with its deep red fruit, within which the tiny nut nestles. This old variety of nut has been consumed by man for thousands of years.

TEACHINGS FROM TIME IMMEMORIAL

❀

The outer shell of the mongongo nut is particularly hard to break. A blow from a stone or the influence of burning embers will crack the armor to reveal a nourishing, protein-rich kernel. The San and Bantu peoples, among many others, used to feast on the pulp of the fruit—whether raw, roasted, or cooked as a porridge. The oil extracted from the mongongo's nut has long been used to enhance and soften dry skin and hair.

ON COLLECTING MONGONGO NUTS

◦

The fruit ripens around April or May, and each female tree bears close to a thousand fruits. The oil that is cold-pressed from the nut is highly stable: it keeps for a long time without going rancid.

THE BENEFITS

◦

The alpha-eleostearic acid which this nut contains forms a particularly efficient protective film around the hair shafts, restoring their vitality. The presence of vitamin A encourages cell turnover and helps to reduce freckles and moles. It is also rich in linoleic acid (omega-6), which protects the skin from external aggressions and has a great ability to prevent dryness. Its high oleic acid content (omega-9) helps alleviate minor cuts and itches.

A FEW DROPS

This oil is potent when it comes to soothing parched skin, but daily application is particularly recommended for the backs of hands that have become patchy from excessively frequent sun exposure. It also protects the neckline area by warding off the onset of brown patches or by helping to alleviate them.

MONGONGO-BASED RECIPES

from Officine Universelle

ANTI–DRY TIPS HAIR MASK

Long hair requires good care: give it a weekly indulgence in the form of this unctuous, nourishing treatment.

Using a bamboo whisk, carefully mix one tablespoon of mongongo oil with two tablespoons of honey and one teaspoon of cider vinegar. Apply along the lengths of the hair down to the tips and leave on for fifteen minutes, then wash with a gentle shampoo and some warm water.

"Why should we plant, when there are so many mongongo nuts in the world?"

BUSHMAN WISDOM

❖ NEEM ❖

Seeds, oil — Origin: India

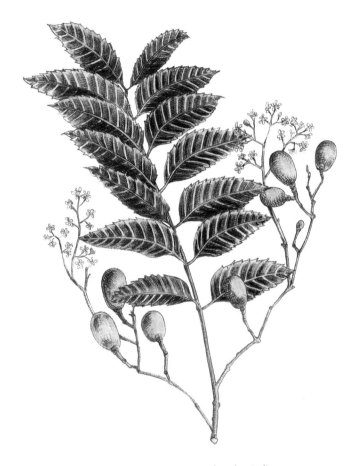

Azadirachta indica

THE ROSARY TREE

*A*zadirachta indica, from the Persian word for "free tree," is native to the dry forests of Deccan and Karnataka in India, as well as Myanmar and Sri Lanka. It has been naturalized in Africa and South America, and is sometimes considered an invasive species. In May, it blooms with clusters of violet flowers, followed by tiny orange fruits upon which birds and bats feed. Often planted along avenues, the tree is reputed to ward off the mosquitoes that transmit malaria. In the

> *"Keep a green tree in your heart and perhaps a singing bird will come."*

CHINESE PROVERB

1990s, neem found itself at the center of an insecticide-focused patent war between the US and India—an emblematic case of bio-piracy. This sort of patenting led to an increase in the price of seeds, which local populations could no longer afford. After ten years spent fighting for the annulment of these patents, traditional Indian medicine won the battle of anteriority.

TEACHINGS FROM TIME IMMEMORIAL

o

Its Sanskrit name means "that which cures all ailments." In Hindu mythology, the tree was born of a drop of amrita, the immortality nectar that fell to Earth during the churning of the sea of milk, at the time of the struggle between the gods and the demons. It is one of the most potent plants in Ayurveda—a quasi-magical panacea. Known as "the village pharmacy," neem is imbued with a variety of properties: the leaves fortify the body against malaria and soothe rheumatism, the fruit is antiparasitic and antiseptic, the twigs and bark are chewed to promote hygiene. The dried leaves, if stored in wardrobes, keep mites away. Tests have shown that some insects would rather die of starvation than bite into its leaves. . . .

ON PREPARING NEEM

o

The neem's kernels are harvested in summer, put out to dry, and crushed in darkness. The process which best preserves their high concentration of active agents is cold-pressing—without chemicals, of course. Neem oil is characterized by its dark brown tint and its scent, which is pungent and spicy, not to mention garlicky and sulfurous, with bitter undertones.

THE BENEFITS

o

Antibacterial, antifungal, anti-inflammatory, insect-repelling . . . neem oil seems to possess limitless virtues, with new ones constantly coming to light, from Ayurveda to the most recent scientific trials. Most of them are attributable to the presence of high concentrations of azadirachtin A. Rich in oleic acid, the oil softens and deeply nourishes the skin.

A FEW DROPS

Neem oil, which is dark and viscous, is applied topically. It can also be diluted in a more fluid oil with a weaker scent. A few drops in your shampoo will fight those invasive parasites that come each school year—headlice. Diluted in another vegetable oil, it will care for the fur of your beloved pets, and rid them of unwanted intruders.

NEEM-BASED RECIPES

from Officine Universelle

DANDRUFF EMERGENCY, OILY AND IRRITATED SCALP

A scalp in disarray will spare you nothing: itches, dandruff . . . Fight back by massaging this oil into the scalp before each shampoo and you'll find lasting peace.

Mix one tablespoon of neem oil, two tablespoons of coconut oil, one drop of cedarwood essential oil, one drop of lavender essential oil, and one drop of rosemary essential oil. Gently heat this mixture in a bain-marie and pour it into a sterilized container. Before shampooing, massage this oil into the scalp, section by section. Leave on for fifteen minutes, then follow with the gentlest possible shampoo. Try gradually spacing out the shampoo sessions once the scalp's flora has been soothed and repaired.

DOWN WITH LICE!

In the merciless struggle between parents and headlice, it's crucial to choose the right weapon. Neem oil, a metal comb, and some conditioner are precious allies.

Cover the whole head of hair with conditioner and run the comb down the length of the hair, section by section and very carefully, wiping the comb clean with paper towels after each stroke. Once face to face with the enemy, you will be able to gauge the severity of the invasion. After running the comb through the entirety of the hair, apply some neem oil (diluted in an equal amount of jojoba oil) to the scalp and the full length of the hair. Leave on for thirty minutes, then shampoo once or twice. Rinsing with vinegar is a must throughout the infestation.

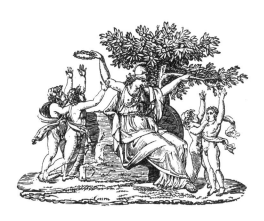

❖ NIGELLA ❖

Oil (seeds) — Origin: Egypt

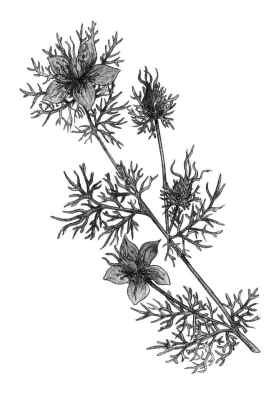

Nigella sativa

A SEED WITH TRUE BLUE FLOWERS

❀

The charming, fresh, pale blue flowers of the nigella bear a fruit whose pod is filled with tiny black seeds, called *niger* in Latin. Acrid and prickly, they are nicknamed "black cumin" or "black caraway," and are highly prized in Indian, Egyptian, and Turkish cuisine. However, this edible nigella, *Nigella sativa*, must not be confused with *Nigella damascena*, which is purely ornamental, or *Nigella arvensis*, whose seeds are toxic.

TEACHINGS FROM TIME IMMEMORIAL

❀

Nigella is an ingredient in ancient remedies, and its essential oil is still used in phytotherapy. Known as *habbat al baraka*, or "blessed seed" in Egypt, nigella's presence in the pharmacopeia has been documented for thousands of years: clay tablets from as far back as the Sumerian civilization bear its name. The Sumerians settled in Mesopotamia on both sides of the Tigris and the Euphrates, a region that was verdant and agricultural at the time.

These tablets, dating back five thousand years, made up a vast repository of some two hundred and fifty plants, including the nigella. Later, on the ancient papyrus discovered at the Luxor archaeological site, which dates back to the 16th century BC, the *Book on the Preparation of Medicine for All Parts of the Human Body* recommended nigella as a cure for pulmonary infections. A vial containing nigella oil was found in Tutankhamen's tomb. Pedanius Dioscorides recommended it to alleviate headaches. In the 11th century, Avicenna, in his *Book of Healing*, devotes an entire chapter to it, praising the seed and its purifying effect. Notably, he encourages crushing it and placing the powder in a purse: inhaling its contents was supposed to help fight the common cold. Islam keeps a special place for it in the pharmacopeia, and upholds it as a panacea.

ON COLLECTING NIGELLA OIL

Once the plant has blossomed, the seeds ripen for a month. From the moment the leaves yellow, the harvest can begin. The green oil obtained by cold-pressing the seeds has a delectable, spicy scent. The essential oil is extracted by hydro-distillation of this vegetable oil.

THE BENEFITS

This precious seed contains more than a hundred different constituents, some of which can't be found anywhere else. Most of the therapeutic benefits of nigella oil can be attributed to thymoquinone, a potent antioxidant, which has been studied for its anticancer properties. Nigelline is the bitter active that stimulates digestion. Nigellone is an anti-allergic substance. Nigella oil is anti-inflammatory and rich in linoleic acid (omega-6), which protects the skin from outside stress and prevents it from drying out. The presence of oleic acid (omega-9) nourishes the skin and helps with the healing of minor scratches and irritations. Vitamin E protects cells from oxidation and carotenoids absorb ultraviolet light.

A FEW DROPS

Nigella oil works wonders on blemishes and small inflammations; it can be applied topically because of its great efficacy. One drop on the affected area purifies the skin, helps it scar over, and improves its appearance.

Since this oil is particularly potent, before using it for the first time, it is recommended to apply one drop on the inside of the wrist and wait fifteen minutes to make sure it is well tolerated.

NIGELLA-BASED RECIPES
from Officine Universelle

UNIVERSAL PURIFYING MASK

By combining the properties of nigella, rhassoul, and lavender, this treatment is a lifesaver for adolescent skin in crisis, and should be added to the whole family's Sunday routine. It regulates excessive sebum production, soothes irritation, and fosters cell renewal.

Mix one tablespoon of nigella oil with one tablespoon of rhassoul and one tablespoon of lavender hydrolate: first pour the oil on the clay, then thin this mixture down with the hydrolate. Gently apply to the face. Leave this mask on for ten minutes. Rinse with warm, clear water, then carefully pat dry with a clean cloth.

FORTIFYING AND STIMULATING OIL FOR THE HAIR

The hair! A common obsession and a harmless pastime. . . . Use the changing of the seasons as an excuse to practice this treatment once or twice a week for a month.

In a three-ounce jar with a dropper, mix three-fifths nigella oil, one-fifth jojoba oil, and one-fifth castor seed oil with ten drops of ylang ylang essential oil for your pleasure. Apply it to the scalp and massage the roots of your hair with the tips of your fingers prior to shampooing. You may also leave this on overnight, with your hair wrapped in a scarf, then wash your hair in the morning.

"The nigella cures everything, except for death."

HADITH

✦ NUT GRASS ✦

Oil (seeds) — Origin: Spain

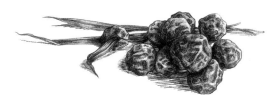

Cyperus esculentus

THE TIGER-STRIPED NUTS

This bright green false weed, which thrives in wetlands and is also known as the "earth almond," produces small, tiger-striped, edible tubers. In Spain they're called *chufa* and considered a delicacy. This invasive species spreads whenever these tubers get stuck to vehicles or other machinery.

TEACHINGS FROM TIME IMMEMORIAL

Nut grass belongs to the noble family of the papyrus. It thrives particularly well on the marshy banks and wide delta of the Nile, and has been found in Egyptian tombs and sarcophagi. Even the ancient Greek physician and botanist Pedanius Dioscorides recommended its tuber to relieve stomach aches. Acclimatized in Spain by Arabic conquerors, its cultivation is particularly intense around Valencia. The Spanish consume its tuber as a plant milk, *horchata de chufa*. In Africa, the seeds located on the plant's flowering tops are crushed to yield a type of flour and a fine oil. In the Maghreb, the oil of this "tiger-striped nut" is reputed to reduce hairiness and promote slow regrowth after waxing in the so-called "Oriental" style, using honey and sugar.

ON COLLECTING THE OIL

Nut grass seeds are harvested twice a year and cold-pressed. The oil is then filtered through a fine cotton cloth. The color of nut grass vegetable oil varies from brown to gold; its scent is easily identifiable, thanks to its light notes of dried fruit.

THE BENEFITS

With its high concentration of oleic acid (omega-9), nut grass oil nourishes the skin and helps injuries scar over. Palmitic acid, a natural emollient, makes it pleasantly supple. Vitamin E (tocopherols) and phytosterols help reduce inflammations. Plants know how to maintain their aura of mystery: though the nut grass's efficient reduction of hairiness has been observed, nothing in its composition would seem to explain this power . . ..

A FEW DROPS

Until the hair liberation movement gets any traction, this oil is known to slow regrowth, and indeed proves very efficient if applied daily on any freshly waxed areas. It also decreases their transitory inflammation and calms the hair's attempts at a precocious regrowth. Very soft to the touch, it makes for a pleasant, hydrating, and soothing oil.

NUT GRASS–BASED RECIPES

from Officine Universelle

AFTERSHAVE TREATMENT

The aftershave is a masculine treatment, but who knows? The art of shaving is not a gendered prerogative. This serum can be applied as often as necessary to slow and soften regrowth.

In a small jar with a dropper, mix one part nut grass oil, one part pomegranate oil, and one part aloe vera gel with five drops of sage essential oil. Applying a few drops to the cheeks, chin, and neck after shaving will soothe razor burn.

POST-WAXING FLUID

Regularly apply this mixture to efficiently reduce irritations, prevent the onset of ingrown hairs, and make regrowth less vigorous.

In a small jar with a dropper, mix one part nut grass oil and one part calendula or marigold oil with fifteen drops of lavender essential oil. Apply to the skin, even if freshly waxed. Massage this oil onto the waxed areas every day for at least a week.

"A fox changes its fur, not its habits."

SUETONIUS

158

❖ OATS ❖

Grains — Origin: Northern Europe

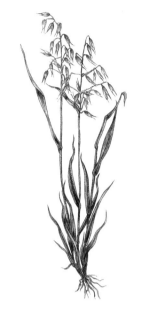

Avena sativa

THE BARBARIANS' BREAD

vena sativa is a grass originating in Northern Europe. Celtic and Germanic peoples used to cultivate it enthusiastically, due to its ability to withstand the rain. To the Romans, it became known as the cereal from which "Barbarians" made bread. Its stem makes for excellent fodder that is especially enjoyed by horses; its cultivation gradually spread throughout Europe along with horse breeding. In the 18th century, as this reputation persisted, the English mocked the Scots for their alleged fondness for oats, despite the fact that the latter only fed them to their horses. Its unpopular and inedible cousin *Avena fatua*, the common wild oat, colonizes cornfields; in French it is nicknamed "the mad oat."

TEACHINGS FROM TIME IMMEMORIAL

This cereal has been cultivated since ancient times and was enhanced through careful selection in the Caucasus and the plains of Turkestan. Its name derives from a Sanskrit word meaning both "sheep" and "food." For Germanic peoples, *loki's hafer*, "the devil's oat," was the name given to grasses that were harmful to cattle and detrimental to the harvest—more likely inspired by the wild oat than by its gentle cousin. Whenever a weed grew in a field, the belief was that Loki, the god of Norse mythology, was there to sow his oats. . . . In the Middle Ages and the Renaissance, physicians and herbalists became a little more interested in the resilience and properties of this banal fodder plant. In 1563, Matthioli wrote that "washing your face with oat flour mixed with white lead will make it beautiful and fair." "When it comes to fighting scabies or infant alopecia, nothing beats bathing in water in which oat straws have been boiled." Oat straws were used for stuffing mattresses as well as healing rheumatism, and according to the French naturopath Jean Valnet, "Children and hotheads would do good to sleep on a mattress made with bales of oat." And when it comes to raising horses, oat has a reputation for making stallions more dashing, but also more rebellious. . . . From beast to man there is but one small step, hence oat's reputation for stimulating male fertility.

ON PREPARING OATS

Two varieties coexist: spring oats and winter oats. The panicles in which the grains are nestled are beaten in order to free the grains. The bran-covered grains can be pressed to make oat flakes. They can also be crushed and sifted to make flour.

THE BENEFITS

Oats are of course recognized for their nutritional values. Used externally, they are emollient, soothing, and purifying. Their proteins and carbohydrates moisturize; their beta-glucan is a polysaccharide with anti-inflammatory and antioxidant properties. Their avenanthramides soothe itches, and their vitamin B stimulates the epidermis.

A FEW PINCHES

Oat is a friend of irritated and intolerant skin; it takes good care of skin that is too tender. Ground to a powder and mixed with water, it can be turned into oat milk, used to gently cleanse the face, or poured into a bath to soothe irritations and itches. As a poultice, it calms the discomfort caused by the dreadful blisters of chicken pox.

OAT-BASED RECIPES
from Officine Universelle

IRRITATION-SOOTHING OAT BATH

The water in our cities is often too hard, and hot baths ill-regarded: splash around in this milky, soothing, and balancing bath, which softens and stimulates the skin.

Using a clean coffee grinder, pulverize 3½ ounces of oat flakes, 1¾ ounces of coarse salt, and 1¾ ounces of chamomile powder, one after the other. Pour those into a fabric sachet and immerse this pouch in a hot bath. Allow to infuse for a few minutes, then dive into the milky bath.

THIRST-QUENCHING MASK FOR DRY HAIR

On a rainy Sunday, take the time to prepare this regenerative mask for hair made dull by winter.

Dilute 1¾ ounces of oat flakes in ¾ cup of warm water, and add one teaspoon of honey and an egg yolk. Mix until you obtain a smooth paste, apply over the whole hair, especially the ends and mid-lengths, and leave on for twenty minutes under a hot towel.

⟡ OLIVE ⟡

Oil (olives) — Origin: Mediterranean basin

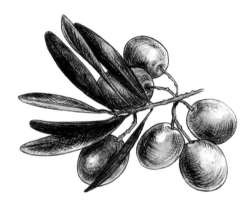

Olea europaea

HOPE

○

With its knotty and grayish trunk, the olive can live for centuries, enduring the aggressions of fire and frost. It has a surprising capacity to regrow from the stump up, out of practically nothing, and then to live and thrive on very little. The stumps of old trees readily emit side shoots that offer them a second youth. No Mediterranean country is complete without a claim to a thousand-year-old olive tree: it is said that Tavira, in Portugal, harbors one that is two thousand years old! The Mediterranean is the "mother" of the olive, which is native to its basin and thrives along its shores. The countries that surround it are the world's primary producers of olives, whose varieties are sorted by usage: table olives, those for oil production, and the versatile ones. Spain is the world's foremost producer of olive oil, and Italy its most avid consumer.

TEACHINGS FROM TIME IMMEMORIAL

○

A symbol of peace and reconciliation for Christians, the olive branch rewarded and crowned winners in the Olympic games of Greek antiquity, while the Quran would later associate the olive with divine light. It was reportedly the Cretans who came up with the idea of extracting its oil by crushing olives with a millstone. Excavations in Knossos, the island's ancient palatial site, have exhumed large ovoid jars of oil dating back two thousand years before our era, and it has been surmised that the tree's cultivation and the crushing of olives were already happening there long before that. Olive oil, which was then considered pure and noble, was burned in Ancient Egypt for the illumination of temples. It was included in the formulation of ointments and balms, while olive leaves were used to cleanse wounds. Greek gymnasts used to anoint themselves with olive oil to care for and highlight their musculature. Long before Marseille built its fortune on the eponymous soap, the town of Aleppo was already thriving thanks to an ancient process of saponification that combined laurel berry oil, olive oil, and plant-based lye. In France, a few olive leaves tucked under a pillow are reputed to make moaners and curmudgeons more affable. In India, olive branches are said to have the capacity to soothe an angry mob . . . .

161

ON COLLECTING OLIVES

◦

The drupes are green and grow darker as they slowly ripen. Between November and January, they are knocked down with a pole and collected in a net hung between the branches. Each tree can yield anywhere from thirty-three to one hundred thirty-two pounds of fruit. Eleven pounds of fruit must be pressed in order to collect one quart of oil, whose color varies from vivid green to pale, greenish yellow. The olives are crushed whole, un-pitted. The resulting mash is then pressed and left to decant to separate the oil from the water. Using a modern centrifuge has now eliminated the associated wait. In order to press a fine oil, time is of the essence: olives must reach the mill on the day they are harvested to prevent any fermentation. The taste and quality of the oil improve for a couple of months, and reach their apex after six months. After two years, the oil starts to oxidize and to lose its taste and properties.

THE BENEFITS

◦

A gentle skin-strengthener: squalenes, of which olive oil packs plenty, are natural components of the epidermis. The antioxidant properties of phenolic compounds, chlorophyll, oleic acid (omega-9) and palmitic acid help hydrate and soothe the skin. Linoleic acid (omega-6) protects it from outside aggressions and efficiently prevents it from drying, while phytosterols activate microcirculation and improve the quality and evenness of the complexion.

A FEW DROPS

Olive oil is without a doubt the most accessible and simply wholesome of natural oils: do not hesitate to apply some sweet and lightly aromatic olive oil to dry skin or hair. You may also resort to soft, beneficial "black soap"—a universal household detergent made of olive oil, salt, and lye. In the olden days, the leaves of olive trees were used as poultices to treat minor wounds; as herbal tea they stimulate our immune system. True goofballs may slather a fine leaf of lettuce in olive oil for a quick, photogenic moisturizing treatment. Leave on for about ten minutes and remove excess oil with a cotton pad soaked with rose water. Your skin is soothed, and you are suddenly as fresh as a green seedling.

"When the dove returned to him in the evening, there in its beak was a freshly plucked olive branch!"

GENESIS 8:11

162

OLIVE-BASED RECIPES

from Officine Universelle

VOLOMANDRA MASSAGE SCRUB

Enjoy the stimulating action of olive pit powder and the vivifying properties of lemon. And go flex your muscles!

In a bowl, mix one tablespoon of olive oil, one level tablespoon of olive pit powder, one heaping tablespoon of yellow clay, and four drops of lemon essential oil. Massage over the whole body (bust and shoulders included) with circular motions. Focus on minor imperfections. Rinse with warm water and pat dry with a towel.

PRETTY GUMS

You take care of your teeth with diligence, and yet your gums are giving you a hard time. Roll up your sleeves and take action.

Pour a small amount of your finest olive oil into a small glass. In the bathroom, after washing your hands and meticulously brushing your teeth, dip a finger into the olive oil and massage your gums for a minute with gentle, circular motions. Use the remaining olive oil for a quick mouthwash; spit it out and rinse with clear water.

To be performed daily until balance is restored.

JUDEA SHAVING OIL

Shaving with a frankincense-boosted oil soothes the razor's burn and heals minors cuts and imperfections. To be used once every three shaves.

Mix two teaspoons of olive oil, two teaspoons of jojoba oil, two teaspoons of oily calendula macerate, one drop of olibanum essential oil, and one drop of myrrh essential oil. Soothe and prepare the skin using a cloth soaked with very hot water (and thoroughly wrung out before use), or simply by running some hot water over your face. Massage the prepared oil into the skin, and shave gently with the grain. Rinse the razor with hot water before each stroke and finish by sprinkling cold water over your face to tighten the pores.

❖ PASSION FRUIT ❖

Oil (seeds) — Origin: Brazil

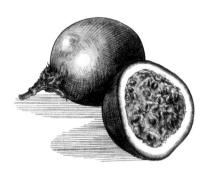

Passiflora edulis

LIANA APPLE

○

This voluptuous, delicious tropical fruit grows on the long lianas of the exotic granadilla. Its exuberantly and delicately designed flowers exude an intoxicating smell. Its name, "passion fruit," reportedly derives from a Guarani word meaning "the fruit that is eaten in one bite." *Maracujá*, in the Tupi language, means "food in a bowl." The first mention of the passion fruit dates back to 1587: the *Descriptive Treatise of Brazil* mentions it as "the fruit-bearing grass." The natural habitat of the four hundred varieties of passion fruit, which the tropical primal forest of South America harbors, is nowadays seriously threatened.

TEACHINGS FROM TIME IMMEMORIAL

○

First spotted in Peru in 1569 by the Spanish physician and botanist Monardes,

in Europe this surprisingly fructiferous *Passiflora* became an ornamental plant, whose flower amazes and seduces.

Legend has it that among an Amazonian tribe, a young girl named Mara, ravishing and glowing, was coveted by all, although she was betrothed to Mamangava, the chief's son. Mad with jealousy, the sorcerer imagined countless charms to conquer her, but it was all in vain. On the eve of the young couple's wedding, he isolated the maiden in the forest, tried and failed to subdue her, and killed her. A distraught Mamangava found her body. At the spot where Mara was buried, a magnificent plant was born. Its flowers were luxuriant, and their scent intoxicating, but it did not bear fruit, as Mara had died a virgin. . . . Mamangava passionately hugged each flower, but each wilted and fell, as the lover himself also wasted away. Mother Nature, finding herself touched, turned Mamangava into a sizable bee, giving him the power to pollinize these extraordinary flowers: their fruit, as sweet as Mara's lips, was called *maracujá*, or "passion fruit."

European botanists were fascinated by its structure. In the 19th century, its chemical composition was analyzed, only to find out that passiflorin reduces anxiety and fosters sleep . . . .

ON PREPARATION

The dozens of seeds and the fleshy, highly aromatic pulp contained in the fruit are cold-pressed: the resulting oil has a fine yellow tint and a discreet fruity scent. It is also called maracujà oil.

ON VIRTUES

Passion fruit oil is rich in vitamin F, which nourishes and embellishes the hair, and in vitamins B2 and B5, which reinforce the hair's structure and foster its growth.

Vitamin E, carotenoids, and bioflavonoids, which the fruit holds in spades, help cells fight oxidative stress. Vitamin K acts on rosacea and redness.

A FEW DROPS

The virtues of this fine oil take natural care of the hair: a few drops, warmed between the palms and worked over the lengths and ends, will work wonders. Redness-prone skin will relish passion fruit oil as a daily moisturizer.

PASSION FRUIT–BASED RECIPES

from Officine Universelle

TREATMENT FOR PERENNIALLY BEAUTIFUL HAIR

Combine the three most highly esteemed hair-care oils to craft a treatment for your hair's weekly maintenance.

In a small jar with a dropper, mix one part passion fruit oil, one part castor seed oil, and one part jojoba oil. Using the dropper, dispense a few drops of this mixture onto the scalp, at the roots of the hair. Massage slowly and work this fluid from the lengths down to the ends. Leave on for at least fifteen minutes under a warm towel, or overnight, and finish with a gentle shampoo.

BRIGHTENING, ANTI-REDNESS FACIAL TREATMENT

Be embarrassed by your rosy cheeks no longer: leave it to this fruity, deliciously scented treatment to tone down their hue.

Using a mortar and pestle, crush the pulp and seeds of a fresh passion fruit along with one small dropper of oil from the same fruit. Slowly rub the resulting paste over the face. Leave on for about ten minutes, then rinse with clear water.

❖ PEARL ❖

Powder — Origin: Tropical seas

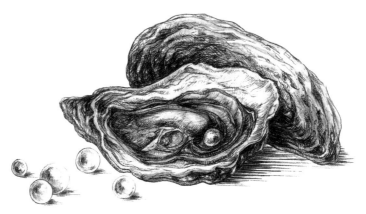

Avicula margaritifera

STAR OF THE SEAS

Pearls are calcareous concretions that form under the nacreous shell and in the soft tissue of certain species of mollusks: cockles, abalones, mussels. . . . The most beautiful ones, which are used for jewelry, are produced by oysters—which, to defend themselves from a foreign body that has entered their shell, secrete a magnificent coating of nacre to envelop the intruder and thus reduce irritation. The mollusk's age and the condition of the seafloor influence the quality of the pearls, their size, and their shine. The beauty of a pearl is appraised based on its shape, size, radiance, and color. Artificially cultured pearls are now much more common than natural ones, which makes for a steady and massive production.

TEACHINGS FROM TIME IMMEMORIAL

The first documented collections or harvests of pearls date back to the third millennium BC. It seems that, since the dawn of time, men have been diving to bring this treasure back up to the surface, braving the danger of the oceans' depths. Pearls are symbols of creation, light, and knowledge. They are miracles of nature, shining expressions of its magic. In the 4th century AD, the theologian Ephrem the Syrian called pearls a "life remedy." According to ancient beliefs, in order to beget a pearl, the oyster comes up to the surface to receive light from the sun or the moon or some heaven-sent fertilizing dew. Born of the sea, the pearl is traditionally dedicated to Aphrodite: much like the Greek goddess of love, it comes from the sea and emerges out of a shell. . . . Alchemists, due to their fascination for transformations and metamorphoses, believed that pearls possessed a power comparable to that of the philosopher's stone. Pearls have always been coveted, pricey jewels, whether as personal adornments or as sacerdotal, royal, or imperial treasures. To this day, certain famous pearls—much like certain diamonds—come with a backstory that is intertwined with the history of great kingdoms or celebrities. So it is with "La Pelegrina," which successively belonged to Mary Tudor, Napoleon III, and Elizabeth Taylor; or "La Régente," which was bought by Napoleon I in 1811. Cleopatra is said to have imbibed a highly valued pearl dissolved in vinegar to enhance her beauty. The radiance of pearls is such that it is reputed to pass to whoever wears one: the pearl thus became a beauty secret. In a section of his memoirs devoted to the preservation of beauty, Sir Kenelm Digby evokes an Eastern custom: "A spoonful of pearl essence—on its own or mixed with two spoonfuls of orange blossom water—is excellent for saving women from the vapors." He also recommends "pearl oil," a complex distillation of pearl powder in vinegar—a recipe that would long remain in vogue. In China, pearls also constitute an ancient remedy and a beauty recipe. Wu Zetian, a powerful Chinese empress

from the 7th century, and Tseu-Hi, a 19th-century regent, consumed pearl powder on a daily basis.

ON PREPARING PEARL POWDER

Pearl powder is obtained from Chinese freshwater-cultured pearls: *Hyriopsis cumingii* and *Cristaria plicata*. The powder's Chinese name is *zhen zu feng*—not to be confused with *zhen zhu mu*, a mediocre powder made from oyster shells. High-quality pearl powder should be white, or have a slight pale-gray tint.

THE BENEFITS

Pearls are naturally made up of calcium carbonate as well as other minerals and trace elements: magnesium, manganese, zinc, and copper. They thus contain more than sixteen amino acids that are greatly beneficial to collagen synthesis and the skin's overall health.

A FEW PEARLS

Wearing pearls boosts the complexion due to the mere proximity of their soft shine: this universal and timeless remedy works for women of all ages. To preserve their beauty, pearls must be worn, for they become dull when stashed away in a box. A pinch of high-quality pearl powder can also be used to beautify a dollop of cream and confer its radiance to your complexion.

⬥ PEONY ⬥

Powder (root) — Origin: China

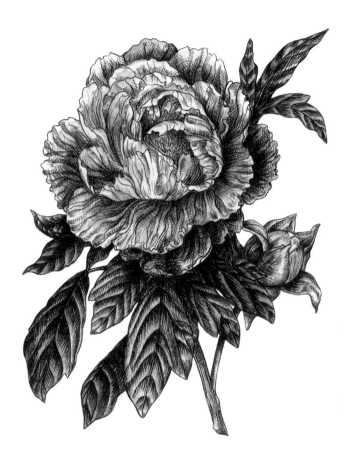

Paeonia suffruticosa, Paeonia rubrae,
and *Paeonia officinalis*

CORAL THRONE

This queen of flowers spreads its petals once a year, and when it blossoms, as brief as it is beautiful, it's a dream to any gardener, painter, or poet. All are seduced by the diversity of its shapes, the graceful and wild opulence of its petals, the subtle variety of its colors and scents. Originating from the Far East—from the woods and prairies of Northern China, Korea, Mongolia, and Japan—its majesty has conquered the whole world with the help of passionate botanists.

TEACHINGS FROM TIME IMMEMORIAL

◉

Paean was the physician of the Olympian gods. He is said to have cured a wounded Hades by administering a peony-based drink. The immodest and flirtatious nymph Peonia was turned into a flower by a jealous goddess (hence the flower's name). Ancient texts show that the Greeks recognized the flower's virtue: around 400 BC, the illustrious physician Hippocrates favored the plant to encourage menstruation as well as the ejection of the placenta following childbirth. In the Middle Ages, peony seed bracelets were said to be imbued with magical and protective properties. The great mystic and healer Hildegarde de Bingen also believed it had the power to dispel fevers. In China, the *mudanhua* is considered a "lucky flower," it symbolizes the renewal of spring and embodies power, nobility and honor. It is often represented alongside a couple of crowing roosters or a phoenix. It was only at the beginning of the Song dynasty (960–1279) that the peony became valued in China, above all for its aesthetic qualities and its subtle scent. It then colonized the ornamentation and gardens of the imperial palaces. In Chinese medicine, the infusion of white peony root powder is highly prized for its ability to heal women by purifying the yin. According to Chinese therapists, "Women who take white peony powder become as beautiful as the flower itself . . ." In 1782, in Hannah Glasse's *The Complete Confectioner*, an English manual for domestic life, the famed cook recommended macerating eighteen fresh peony roots seasoned with herbs, flowers, and spices in a gallon of spirit wine to treat "all nervous disorders."

One can also follow the French dictum: *"Take the blooming peony, put it under your pillow, and in your sleep you will dream of happiness."*

ON COLLECTING PEONY ROOTS

◉

Peony roots are harvested (i.e., uprooted) by hand. The knots are removed and the roots are meticulously washed, dried, and crushed to a powder.

THE BENEFITS

◉

The peony has a regenerative effect upon the skin. Paeoniflorin is a potent natural anti-irritant with soothing, antiradical, and anti-inflammatory properties. The peony encourages circulation and helps care for mature skin.

A FEW PINCHES

What a delight it is to sprinkle one's beauty products with ravishing pink peony powder, in order to harness its calming properties. Over the course of a month, one teaspoon of powder in a hair mask or a gentle shampoo will soothe sensitive and irritated scalps. . . . Combined with an equal amount of very fine iris root powder, it makes for a perfect dry shampoo.

PEONY-BASED RECIPES

from Officine Universelle

SOOTHING AND RESTORATIVE PEONY MASK

Springtime is here; the time of plunging necklines and summer dresses has arrived. This rebirth will make you crave this toning and softening flowery preparation.

In a small bowl, carefully mix together two tablespoons of peony powder, one tablespoon of white clay, and three tablespoons of rose water with five drops of rose hip seed oil. Apply this mask to the chest—and, if you feel like it, all the way up to the neck and face. Leave on until the mask starts to harden. Rinse with clear lukewarm water. Pat dry with a spotlessly clean cloth.

COMFORTING BATH

A handful of peony salts will give your bath a delightful scent and soothe your spirit. If the flower is in season, add some fresh petals to your hot bath.

Before bathing, mix one tablespoon of peony powder, three tablespoons of coarse salt, two tablespoons of oats, and three drops of orange blossom essential oil together in a bowl. Add to the bathwater before you step in.

"From the peony's heart
The bee exits
With such regret!"

MATSUO BASHŌ (1644–94)

✤ PERILLA ✤

Oil and essential oil, grains — Origin: Southeast Asia

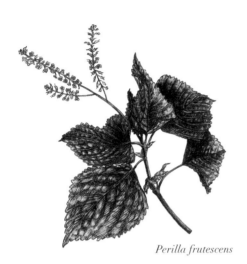

Perilla frutescens

WILD SESAME

○

This aromatic plant, whose prized leaves are used as condiments, is highly sought-after throughout Asia: *kaetip* in Korea, *shiso* in Japan, *zi-su* in China. The taste of its tiny black seeds is comparable to that of sesame; its leaves, bright green to purple in color, have a distinctive aroma—both herbaceous and deliciously acidulous. Perilla is native to mountainous regions and is identifiable by its serrated, downy leaves; it thrives from the Himalayas to Myanmar. Japanese immigrants imported it to the United States: perilla was then nicknamed the "beefsteak plant," as it was used to simultaneously flavor and preserve beef. In Korea and Japan, this delightful herb is one of the ingredients of fermented preparations such as kimchi and umeboshi.

TEACHINGS FROM TIME IMMEMORIAL

○

In China, in the 6th century, the various uses of perilla seeds and leaves were already being mentioned in the medicine treatise *Ming Yi Bie Lu*, by the Taoist monk Tao Hong-Jing, the Huayang hermit. The seeds help fight persistent coughs, tame asthma, hiccups, and fatigue. The leaves alleviate headaches and help treat the flu and food-borne intoxications. In Japan, perilla leaves often find a culinary pairing with shellfish or the perilous *fugu*, the Japanese fish that is toxic if not prepared properly. Nowadays, in Asia, perilla's protective action against allergic reactions is spurring scientific studies, which have confirmed the validity of this use. As the correspondent of the "King's garden" in China, the Jesuit Pierre d'Incarville, who lived in Beijing from 1740 to 1757, sent perilla seeds back to his botany professor Pierre de Jussieu in France, thereby introducing the plant into Europe.

ON COLLECTING WILD SESAME

○

The tiny seeds of perilla are cold-pressed to yield a fine oil that has the aroma of pencil lead and is highly sensitive to oxidation: it must be kept refrigerated after opening. Distilling the fresh leaves of perilla allows for the extraction of an herbaceous-scented essential oil.

THE BENEFITS

Perilla oil has a particularly high concentration of fatty acids. Its high concentration of alpha-linoleic acid (omega-3) strengthens its soothing action, encourages the hydration and regeneration of skin cells and the scarification process, and minimizes inflammatory phenomena. The essential oil, made up of more than 50% aldehydes, is a potent antioxidant with antifungal and antibacterial properties, which fights free radicals and tonifies the organism.

A FEW DROPS

This still largely unsung vegetable oil helps both irritated and mature skin: daily use will provide swift and visible comfort. Massaged topically, it helps soothe rheumatic pain. For increased efficiency, it is possible to mix 5% perilla essential oil into 95% perilla vegetable oil, which will also help it to keep for longer.

PERILLA-BASED RECIPES

from Officine Universelle

"THREE CONTINENTS, THREE CURES" OIL

For dry or damaged skin, or a creased complexion, use this at any given moment . . . the soothing, healing, and antiaging properties of this fluid will work wonders.

In a small two-ounce jar with a dropper, mix one part perilla oil, one part sea buckthorn oil, one part rose hip seed oil, and three drops of patchouli essential oil.

"With the scent of bluish shiso my heart is purified."

KADOTA ASAHI

PINK SAKE LOTION

The virtues of seeing "la vie en rose" no longer need to be demonstrated: purifying and softening, this felicitous lotion for combination or oily skin combines the benefits of sake and umeboshi.

Rinse eight umeboshi plums in clear, hot water, then put them in a bowl and cover them with water. Let them sit for two days, changing the water several times so as to remove any trace of salt. Add the eight desalted plums to a small bottle of sake and allow to macerate for a week. Filter the preparation into another bottle. It will keep for up to a month in the fridge. It is to be applied nightly to the face, using a cotton pad.

✣ POMEGRANATE ✣

Natural oil (pomegranate seeds) — Origin: Turkey

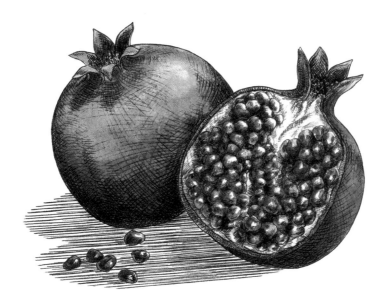

Punica granatum

IN SOLOMON'S ORCHARDS

॰

The pomegranate is the most frequently cited fruit in the Bible, as well as one of the blessed fruits of Buddhism. King Solomon had plenty of pomegranates planted in his orchards. Celebrated in numerous religions and myths as a token of prosperity and fertility, the pomegranate's fleshy arils (bright red seeds nestled at the core of the fruit) symbolize bright days in the East and on all Mediterranean shores. The pomegranate's Roman name refers to the Carthaginian civilization; this "Punic apple" was also an emblem of the city, because of its guardian goddess,

Tanit Punica. As is often the case, it was reportedly the Phoenicians who first imported this fruit from Iran. After a reddish-orange blossoming, in the autumn this evergreen sprouts soft fruit that can be sweet or bitter depending on the type.

TEACHINGS FROM TIME IMMEMORIAL

॰

It is said that the Anatolian mother goddess Cybele was impreganted by a pomegranate set atop her womb. The Assyrian love goddess Ishtar is often represented clasping a pomegranate. As for the hadiths, they report that "There is no pomegranate that does not carry a pomegranate seed from heaven." On Renaissance paintings depicting the Madonna and Child, the Infant Jesus is often seen holding a pomegranate. Its ruby-colored seeds and the vermilion juice that flows from them make it a symbol of life and passion, of love and resurrection. Favored by caravan drivers, protected from drying out by its thick skin, the restorative pomegranate quenches thirst and heals. Its bark has been used as a dewormer since Ancient Egyptian times, where the fruit was also found in tombs, by the side of the noble individuals interred there. Its juice and seeds are reputedly purifying, fortifying, and conducive to digestion.

ON COLLECTING POMEGRANATE SEED OIL

o

A recent, highly technical and heatless extraction method is nowadays used to extract all the benefits from these miraculous seeds. This ecological process, which does not involve any petrochemical solvent, is CO_2 extraction: it enables the production of highly concentrated extracts of great purity that are faithful to the original plant. Subjected to an extremely high level of compression, the gas liquefies and becomes a solvent of the active ingredients it traverses. The pressure is then lowered and the gas, once again unstable, is captured in order to be recycled and reused. The oil thus obtained has a rather fine and light texture, along with a pale yellow tint and a very discreet fragrance that simultaneously evokes fruit and cookies.

THE BENEFITS

o

Pomegranate seed oil contains a very high concentration of alpha-punicic acid (omega-5), an essential fatty acid with a high antioxidant potency, which is found exclusively in this seed. The phytosterols it contains help reduce inflammation.

It is also very rich in oleic acid (omega-9) and linoleic acid (omega-6), which nourish the epidermis and foster cell turnover. It stimulates the skin's self-repair mechanisms.

"In a pomegranate garden, the fruits looked like earthen pots. He took a few, and no sooner had he opened them that birds of the prettiest colors came out of them and flew away."

THE ROSE OF BAKAWALI, LEGEND

A FEW DROPS

A benefactor of sensitive skin types, pomegranate seed oil is anti-inflammatory, soothing, and potently antioxidant. It should be used directly on damaged or mature skin. It is also a gentleman's ally when it comes to alleviating razor burn, and a lifesaver for summer vacationers since it expertly soothes sunburn.

POMEGRANATE-BASED RECIPES

from Officine Universelle

INSTANT BEAUTY RECOVERY MASK

Do you believe in the virtue of pink, both in your wardrobe and on your cheeks? This autumn mask brings you radiance and color.

Blend together two tablespoons of seeds from a well-ripened and fresh pomegranate with a spoonful of honey and one of rose water. Use gloves and be careful not to stain your clothes. Apply, avoiding the eye area, and leave on for fifteen minutes.

GREAT QUICK SCRUB

Regularly scrubbing your face, as long as you don't overdo it (say, once a week to once every ten days), is the best way to care for your skin's grain and the freshness of your complexion.

Carefully mix together one teaspoon of pomegranate seed oil, one tablespoon of iris root powder, and five tablespoons of verbenone rosemary hydrolate. Slowly massage the resulting paste on the face, forehead, and neck, as well as the sides of the nose, and rinse with clear, warm water.

❖ PRACAXI ❖

Oil (seeds) — Origin: Brazil

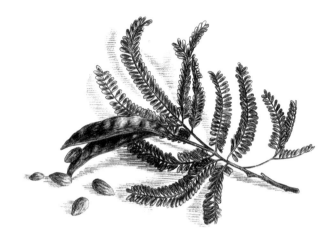

Pentaclethra macroloba

RESOURCEFUL ROOT

○

A scion of the Fabaceae family, this breed of mimosa looks somewhat like a palm tree. The pracaxi thrives in the humid areas of northern South America and in Central America. Its impressive growth rate and its capacity to capture nitrogen through its roots help deeply enrich and quickly regenerate the depleted soils of the most devastated forests.

TEACHINGS FROM TIME IMMEMORIAL

○

For thousands of years, the crushed bark of the tree has been used as a plaster by Amerindians to combat the effects of snake bites and scorpion stings. They also use its oil to fight skin infections, notably erysipelas. In Amazonia, people treat their hair with the oil extracted from pracaxi

seeds so as to ward off its loss, make it easier to tame, and enhance its shine. Pregnant women apply it to prevent the onset of and minimize stretch marks.

ON PREPARATION

○

The pracaxi's pretty, half-moon-shaped pods hold a few seeds which are harvested from December to March. When ripe, their color changes from green to dark brown. The harvest must be performed directly on the tree, before the fruit opens, but not before it has matured fully. The fruits must be transported in raffia bags so as to stay protected from the sun. The pods are dried in the shade and the seeds are extracted manually. Traditionally, they used to be roasted and later crushed using a mortar in order to extract the precious oil. Forty or so pods will hold about two pounds of seeds, which are made up of about 33% oil, whose color varies from deep yellow to brown. Its scent is reminiscent of peanuts and humus.

ON VIRTUES

Pracaxi oil boasts the highest concentration of behenic acid, a rare acid whose properties help tame and treat the hair and scalp. Oleic acid (omega-9) and palmitic acid help hydrate and mollify the skin. Lignoceric acid gives the oil its lightness and its impressive capacity to be absorbed. Its phytosterols activate microcirculation, while its vitamin E reduces inflammation and protects the cells from oxidation.

A FEW DROPS

The most common cosmetic use of pracaxi consists in embellishing the hair: applied directly, this fine, readily absorbed oil takes control of curly hair and minimizes frizzing. Applied as a mask on the scalp, it soothes it and helps ward off hair loss. It is also suitable to pacify damaged skin and to reduce depigmentation marks and smooth out patchy skin.

PRACAXI-BASED RECIPES

from Officine Universelle

The most common cosmetic use of pracaxi consists in embellishing the hair: applied directly, this fine, readily absorbed oil takes control of curly hair and minimizes frizzing. Applied as a mask on the scalp, it soothes it and helps ward off hair loss. It is also suitable to pacify damaged skin and to reduce depigmentation marks and smooth out patchy skin.

MIRACLE TREATMENT FOR PATCHY HANDS AND NECKLINES

In a three-ounce jar with a dropper, mix one part pracaxi oil and one part castor seed oil with seven drops of geranium essential oil. Apply this mixture after summer, when your suntan has faded away, on the face, the neckline area, and the backs of your hands.

PRESERVING, ANTI–HAIR LOSS SERUM

In a jar with a dropper, mix one part pracaxi oil and one part tamanu oil. Massage this mixture on the roots of the hair, all over the front of the scalp. Leave on for a night under a scarf, or for half an hour. Finish with a gentle shampoo, and rinse carefully.

⟡ PRICKLY PEAR ⟡

Oil (pips) — Origin: Morocco

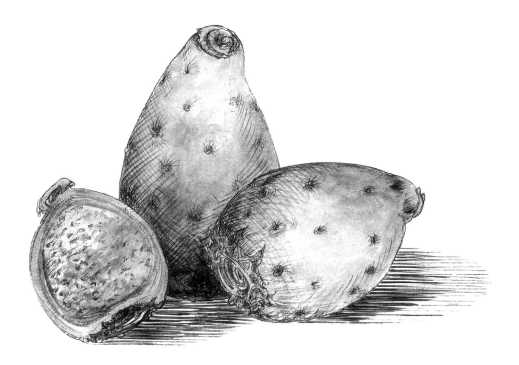

Opuntia ficus indica

UNDER THE THORNS, THE MIRACLE PLANT

○

Native to South America and acclimatized in the wake of Christopher Columbus, *Opuntia ficus indica* is an arborescent cactus. Its stem is made up of fleshy, thorny paddles whose extremities sprout orange flowers followed by ovoid fruits covered in tiny,

stubborn barbs: the prickly pears. Once peeled (carefully, because of the spines), the yellow- to coral-tinted pulp is edible and delicious. It is shot through with tiny dark pips that hold the plant's oil. *Ficus indica* has been grown for more than five thousand years by Amerindian peoples, especially in Mexico. Nicknamed "the Christian's fig" by the Arabs, its generous and providential fruit, rich in fibers and vitamins, contributes to the nutritional balance of numerous populations to this day.

TEACHINGS FROM TIME IMMEMORIAL

◦

This delicious fruit-bearing cactus was unknown in Europe and Africa before the voyages of Christopher Columbus. *Ficus indica* gained a foothold thanks to trade and the Spanish conquest, and slowly colonized the whole Mediterranean basin until it became an essential part of the landscape, from Morocco to Southern Italy and Greece. In the Americas during the pre-Columbian era, *nopal* — the Aztec name for the cactus — was primarily grown to enable the farming of female cochineals. This tiny insect, which has a particular taste for this type of cactus, was prized for its high concentration in bright red pigment, which made it possible to color textile fibers a deep, radiant, and highly durable red. In traditional Aztec medicine, prickly pear poultices were used to cure rheumatism and broken bones, and its juice was used to soothe burns. In Morocco, where this cactus thrives splendidly, its fruit pulp soothes the skin after a long day spent working in the fierce, havoc-wreaking sun.

ON COLLECTING PRICKLY PEAR OIL

◦

Patience is the name of the game when extracting the oil because the tiny seeds that dot the pulp of the fruit are only 5% oil. Harvesting and seeding 1,765 pounds of prickly pears, followed by rinsing,

drying, and cold-pressing their pips, only yields one humble quart of oil. Precious and expensive, this pale yellow oil has a very discreet spicy scent. Prickly pear flower macerate is full of benefits, but less effective than the plant's natural oil.

THE BENEFITS

◦

The myth that presents prickly pear oil, not unreasonably, as an elixir of youth is due to its high concentration of sterols, tocopherols, and tocotrienols — vitamin E — which help protect against free radicals and improve microcirculation within the skin. Linoleic acid — omega-6 — increases cell turnover. All these virtues combine to make prickly pear oil a natural antiaging and skin-tightening treatment.

A FEW DROPS

The highly precious prickly pear oil is the rarest and most expensive of oils. You have to be old enough to deserve it! A few drops on your face and chest in the evening will be enough to ensure a potent youth-preserving effect, provided it is applied regularly.

PRICKLY PEAR–BASED RECIPES

from Officine Universelle

SOFTENING
PRICKLY PEAR PULP MASK

An experiment for beauty adventuresses, those who feel galvanized by difficulties and who like to boast of their exploits.

Don gloves and peel the tenacious and thorny skin off a well-ripened prickly pear. Mash the pulp with a fork. Add two tablespoons of yogurt to the fruit and blend thoroughly until you get an even mixture. Place a fine sheet of gauze over your face (an unfolded bandage will do the trick) and apply this mask. Leave on for about ten minutes, then remove the mask by lifting the gauze and rinse with warm water.

POTENT ANTIAGING SERUM

Just because you like to do as little as possible doesn't mean you don't care about appearances: this combination of three oils most valuable to mature skin was made for you.

In a small jar with a dropper, mix 50% prickly pear oil, 25% argan oil, and 25% açaí oil. A few drops applied nightly on the face, neck, and neckline area will work wonders, and replace many a complex treatment, especially after exposure to the sun in the summer.

"You only realize the value of something when it becomes rare."

MOROCCAN PROVERB

⚜ RASPBERRY ⚜

Seeds, oil — Origin: Turkey

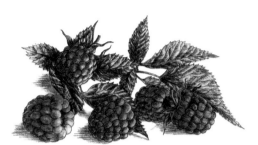

Rubus idaeus

THE DELICIOUS BRAMBLE

○

The raspberry bush, a wild shrub that has acclimatized everywhere from the Arctic polar circle to the tropics, produces abundant fruit that is as virtuous as it is tasty. The *Rubus* genus seems to originate from Asia Minor, a region which roughly corresponds to present-day Turkey. Pliny the Elder was the first to describe this bush, with its delicious berries and creeping branches covered in defensive thorns, and to give it a name: "Mount Ida bramble." Grown in Europe since Roman times, the species was domesticated to improve the size and flavor of its berries, which we usually picture as red but which can also be white, black, or even yellow!

TEACHINGS FROM TIME IMMEMORIAL

○

It is said that a young Zeus was having a crying fit when the nymph Ida gave him a delicious berry—a raspberry—to calm him down. But as she was picking it, the fair nymph pricked her bosom, tinting the white berry with her ruby-colored blood. Its benefits are recognized by all the far-flung peoples that make it part of their diet. In Europe, it is alleged that the branches of wild raspberry bushes, when hung outside a house, will protect its inhabitants. In North America, raspberries were preserved in fat by Amerindians and used to fight infections as well as the flu. In the 18th century, the Irish herbalist K'Eogh wrote about the raspberry: "An application of honey and crushed flowers will treat the eye's inflammations . . . the fruit is good for the heart."

ON COLLECTING RASPBERRY SEED OIL

○

The highly fragile and delicate berries are harvested between June and September. A raspberry bush will bear fruit for a decade. The seeds are separated from the pulp, dried, crushed, and cold-pressed to obtain a blond-colored oil with a fruity, fresh, and light smell.

THE BENEFITS

○

Raspberry seed oil takes care of skin that has been damaged by sun and the cold. It is made up of about 50% linoleic acid—omega-6—which fosters cell regeneration, prevents the skin from drying out, and helps reconstitute epidermal lipids. Its high concentrations of alpha-linolenic acid—an omega-3—vitamin E, gallic acid, and carotenoid help prevent cellular decay.

A FEW DROPS

Raspberry seed oil can be applied at night directly to a thoroughly, but always gently, cleansed face. It is very rapidly absorbed and does wonders to ward off redness, dryness, and the signs of aging.

RASPBERRY-BASED RECIPES

from Officine Universelle

GENTLE RASPBERRY SEED OIL FACIAL EXFOLIANT

This treatment—part mask, part scrub— evens out the complexion and soothes the epidermis. A nighttime ritual to give your skin a makeover.

In the palm of your hand or in a small bowl, mix two tablespoons of raspberry seed oil, two drops of chamomile essential oil, and one tablespoon of wheat or white clay. Gently rub the mixture on your face, particularly on the areas whose grain you wish to refine. Rinse with warm water and pat dry with a soft cloth.

RASPBERRY FACIAL CLEANSING MILK

With the return of summer comes the pleasure of preparing this cleansing treatment, which will delight all pink aficionados. Be generous with your cosmetic creations, and share them with your loved ones. Where there's enough for one mask, there's enough for two. . . .

Blend a dozen fresh raspberries along with three tablespoons of powdered organic milk and a small amount of floral water. Cleanse your face with the resulting paste, spreading it with little circular motions. Rinse. Pat dry with a soft cloth and enjoy your newfound smoothness.

⊹ RICE ⊹

Oil, bran, flour, and vinegar (grains) — Origin: Asia

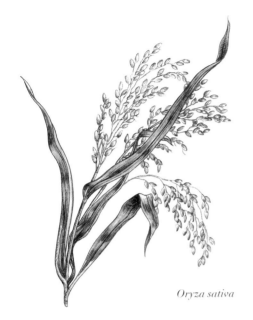

Oryza sativa

GO WITH THE GRAIN

Oryza sativa is one of the plants most useful to mankind: it produces the rice grain. One of the cradles of the cultivation of rice is Southern China, as early as the fifth century BC. Among the twenty-odd known species, *indica* and *japonica* are the most common. There are about 130,000 varieties of rice, half of which are still cultivated. This cereal, consumed almost solely by humans, is mostly cultivated in tropical Asian countries, usually by small producers. Its cultivation gradually spread throughout the world. This herbaceous, vigorous cereal grows with its toes in the water, and is not fussy about soil quality. It thrives on the same plots of land for decades, or even centuries. Rice's cultivation in flooded paddy fields gives birth to spectacular, magnificent agricultural landscapes, some of which are terraced down the slopes of tall hills. Rice, which nourishes a significant share of the world's population, is very labor-intensive to grow. The method of transplantation makes it possible to harvest twice a year.

TEACHINGS FROM TIME IMMEMORIAL

Rice has always been a symbol of life and plenty in Eastern civilizations. In India, the sowing of rice is preceded by a ceremony: priests ask the gods to intercede in favor of a felicitous harvest. Each year in China, the emperor would perform a religious ritual during which he would plant a rice tree with his own hands. Good fortune and favorable omens rain down on newlyweds along with the rice thrown upon them by their guests at the end of the ceremony. Rice is also a symbol of fertility: holding some rice in hand will bring the bride happiness and motherhood. . . . Numerous legends in many cultures and societies illustrate the importance that is bestowed upon rice. In India, a local legend tells the story of Saint Thomas turning grains of sand into rice to feed the workers who were building his church. In Laos, a tale tells of the sorrow the grain of rice feels

> *"A spoonful of rice when you're hungry is better than a bushel of rice when you're full."*

GEORGES CLÉMENCEAU

when it is left alone. In Japan, Inari, god of rice, and his messenger, the fox, are worshiped. In China, rice is the first star in the constellation devoted to the cereals. In traditional Chinese medicine, rice is a neutral food; it "fortifies the body and gives one a fine appearance." In Europe, its first cosmetic use was in the famed rice powder: as early as the late 19th century, people would "powderize" themselves at every opportunity to obtain a matte complexion. In Japan, water that is used to rinse rice, or *yu-su-ru*, is collected and stored so it can be applied to the hair, which it protects. Rice bran, or *nuka*, has for centuries been a beauty secret—a gentle exfoliant that cleanses, purifies, and brightens the complexion.

ON PREPARING RICE

The panicles of rice are harvested and brought to the rice mill for sorting. The rice grain is made up of the endosperm, the germ, and the coat (or bran). Most of rice's nutritional value is concentrated in the latter. In its full, unhusked form, rice is known as paddy. When rid of its first envelope, the husk, it becomes brown rice; remove the bran and you get white rice. The bran is obtained by mechanical

abrasion of brown rice. Rice bran oil is obtained by pressing the envelope of brown rice. It has a pale tint and a gentle scent. Rice vinegar is obtained by acetic fermentation of rice wine, or sake, which is obtained from white rice that has been further polished with water.

THE BENEFITS

Rice bran oil is a sure source of vitality for the skin. The numerous enzymes it contains protect the skin from aging. Rice has a high concentration of antioxidants—oryzanols, vitamin E—and mineral salts that are indispensable to the proper functioning of the epidermis; it is also rich in phytosterols and carotenoids, which help soothe and calm irritated skin.

A FEW PINCHES OR A FEW DROPS

For city-dwellers who wish to help their skin fight pollution and stress, rice bran oil is a panacea. It protects the skin and fights oxidation as well as the signs of aging. Whenever you cook quality organic white rice, rinse it and keep the water as a precious commodity: it is ideal for rinsing the hair. Frozen into ice cubes, it can also stimulate microcirculation, alleviate the bags under your eyes, and care for dry lips. Rice flour masks are excellent as a way to calm down skin inflammation.

RICE-BASED RECIPES

from Officine Universelle

RICE BELLE

This soothing mask is an ideal weekly ritual for restoring balance to intolerant skin and caring for mature skin.

Mix a heaping 2½ teaspoons of rice flour with five heaping teaspoons of rice bran, adding a little warm water infused with floral water. Apply the resulting paste to your (well-cleansed) face and leave on for about ten minutes. Gently rinse with warm water and pat dry thoroughly with a spotlessly clean cloth.

ALABASTER COMPLEXION

Avoid the sun's rays that age the skin prematurely and harness rice's virtues to care for your dovelike complexion.

Fill a very fine, small cotton bag with rice bran. Plunge it into a very hot bath. Once the bath has cooled down to your preferred temperature, step into the water (you must have cleansed yourself beforehand); run the sachet at length over your face, neck, and neckline area. Get out of the bath without rinsing and pat dry.

RICE VINEGAR SUMMER BATH

Make peace with high temperatures and the surrounding dampness and reconnect with the joy of being active on the warmest days: dive into a toning and softening bath.

Pour two large tumblers of brown rice vinegar into a tub filled halfway with lukewarm water: step into the bath (when already clean) and remain in there for about ten minutes. Do not rinse—just pat yourself dry.

TANNING RICE-BASED SCRUB

A great miracle scrub, to be used once a month to carry the radiance of your summer body into the winter.

Combine half a cup of ground brown rice (with the texture of a coarse flour), half a cup of organic coconut milk, half a cup of grated organic coconut, and a tablespoon of ground turmeric in a blender: once the mixture has become smooth, massage vigorously over the whole body, using circular motions, for a good five minutes. Remove the excess paste with a natural sponge, then rinse with warm water.

✦ ROSE ✦

Flower, water, powder, oil — Origin: Central Asia

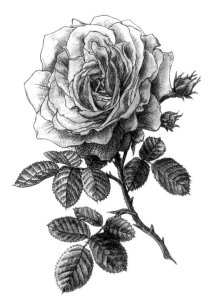

Rosa damascena, Rosa gallica,
and *Rosa rubiginosa*

A FLOWER FROM
THE DAWN OF TIME

Originating in Central Asia, the Rosacea family has spawned countless species that either hybridized naturally or were multiplied by man. Its prolific bushes all descended from an original wild rosebush, *Rosa canina*, whose diminutive flowers number five petals, much like the elegant sweet briar dotting the countryside. Among its offspring, *Rosa damascena*, *Rosa gallica*, and *Rosa rubiginosa* are the three variations whose flowers are most commonly used in beauty treatments.

THE ROMANCE OF THE ROSE

The Greeks dedicated the rose to Aphrodite, while for the Christians it was Mary. According to myth, the goddess of love stained a white rosebush with her blood, thus giving birth to red roses. From the gardens of Midas to the baths of Roman *thermae*, from Cleopatra's bed to Marie-Antoinette's Trianon, through their beauty and their fragrance, roses have bewitched women, men, heroes, and the gods alike.

Before it became ornamental, the rose was first and foremost medicinal and sacred: temples are washed with its water; Charlemagne encouraged its cultivation near religious buildings so that its properties could be studied and spread. Evidence has shown that rose water was widely traded in the Middle East in the 9th century: it has been attested that thirty thousand bottles of this elixir were delivered from the Faristan Province in Iran to Baghdad in Iraq. In the 13th century, the Provins Rose, or *Rosa gallica* 'Officinalis,' was nicknamed the "apothecary's rose." It was an efficient addition to the ingredients of skin ointments and remedies. Highly sought after, it has become a symbol for the ephemeral quality of beauty in most of the cultures in which it grows. Ronsard, Shakespeare, Apollinaire: all the poets have celebrated its beauty, which stands as a metaphor for love and of time's flight. Today, the rose is still a revered beauty secret.

ON HARVESTING ROSES

◦

The flower, which comes in a variety of shapes, colors, and fragrances, can be distilled to obtain rose water or essential oil. The buds and petals are harvested to be simply dried or crushed to a powder, while the seeds of *Rosa rubiginosa* are cold-pressed to extract rose hip seed oil, a precious, highly fragrant vegetable oil with potent properties. Roses must be plucked by hand at dawn, at six o'clock, when the fragrance of the flower, replete with morning dew, is at its finest. Once harvested in this manner, the flowers are distilled on the same day to ensure that wilting does not allow their properties to spoil. The steam, laden with aromatic compounds, naturally separates from   the essential oil at the mouth of the alembic's exit spout, before condensing into rose water.

Before they are crushed to a powder, the petals are left to dry in the open air for several days. Avoid spraying pesticides or chemical treatments onto the roses in your garden—you will then be able to pluck the petals of your finest flowers before they bloom too widely and turn them into a fine powder that can be stored in a dry place. The seeds of the Chilean "musk rose" are harvested at the foot of the Andes, and its fruits are dried in the sun— or in low-temperature ovens—using a gentle heat. The seeds are crushed, sieved, and gently cold-pressed.

ON SELECTION

◦

Fine rose water is colorless. Its fragrance is that of the flower, but remains very mild and ephemeral. Its scent should be light and fresh. Rose water must be stored in an airtight container in a cabinet, away from direct sunlight. A good rose powder or dried rose petals should be chosen based on the intensity of their color and on their fragrance. The more vivid the tint and the scent, the higher the concentration in active ingredients. Rose hip seed oil naturally boasts a very bright orange hue. Its vegetable oil fragrance, gently oily, should be discreet.

THE BENEFITS

◦

Rose water and rose oil are the most ancient remedies to ward off the signs of aging and boost skin tone, as they are notably highly concentrated in vitamins C and E. Dull, tired skin as well as mature and lifeless skin will savor their high concentration of essential fatty acids, which protect against free radicals. They help fight skin aging, smooth out even the most fragile skin or the finest areas, and tone it up. Damask rose petal powder is a great classic of Ayurvedic medicine, which prescribes it for the care of sensitive, weakened, and mature skin. High in astringent tannins, it gently refines the skin's grain and tightens its pores. Highly concentrated in rose oil, gallic acid is a well-documented antioxidant, and linoleic acid (omega-6) protects the skin from exposure, nourishing it and preventing it from drying out. Alpha-linolenic acid (omega-3) and pro-vitamin A foster the process of skin cell regeneration.

A FEW DROPS
OF ROSE WATER AND OIL

Rose water is *the* indispensable lotion in skincare, a classic that no bathroom could do without. Its ease of use and efficacy mean that it should be turned to daily, for perfect facial cleansing at night or to awaken the skin in the morning, using a cotton pad or a spray for a soft finish. Sprayed onto the scalp, it fortifies fine and fragile hair by boosting microcirculation and thus fostering growth. Applying rose hip seed oil before you step out the door will boost your complexion. Gently and directly massaged on the face just before bedtime, it heals dry skin and works wonders when applied topically on a scar or burn, or over the whole body, notably to assist with healing stretch marks.

A FEW PETALS

Pluck the petals off your roses; they are precious and can be used in a variety of treatments. Steeped directly in a warm bath, fresh rose petals lead to relaxation and a lifting of the spirits.

For an invigorating and purifying steam bath, lay out fresh petals on a sieve resting on a container filled with boiling water. Expose your face to the steam for a few minutes—it gets loaded with fragrance and active ingredients as it rises through the petals: what a delight!

Dried and crushed to a powder, then mixed with a little tepid water and a few drops of rose hip seed oil, they make for a gentle, stimulating scrub suitable for all skin types.

ROSE-BASED RECIPES

from Officine Universelle

ROSE VINEGAR

Scented vinegars are an ancient and highly effective way of polishing skin and scalp care. It is a quaint treatment—but one that has proved its worth.

After plucking a few just-bloomed flowers early one morning in your garden, or using rosebuds procured from a reputable herbalist, steep 3½ ounces of their petals for fifteen days in one quart of white wine vinegar, which you will have previously brought to a boil. Filter the brew and marvel at its sumptuous pink color. This lotion will keep for a month in a glass bottle stored away from sunlight. Use after shampooing to rinse and lend shine to the hair, or on a cotton pad to purify the skin's complexion.

RADIANT FACIAL BOOST

The ultimate classic for normal, sensitive, or dry skin: a lifelong weekly treatment.

In a small bowl, mix one level tablespoon of rose petal powder, one teaspoon of apricot kernel oil, and a scant tablespoon of rose water. Work the mixture into a soft paste and gently rub onto the face and neck. Rinse with warm water and softly pat the face dry with a spotlessly clean cloth.

"BRIGHT EYES AND CLEAR SKIN" TREATMENT

Rose water's properties are enhanced by cold temperatures. Well-organized types can experience the joy of keeping these miraculous ice cubes in the freezer.

Freeze some rose water in a spotlessly clean ice cube tray. To reduce the rings, bags, and swelling that accompany tired eyes, and to give one's general appearance a welcome boost, slowly run a rose water ice cube wrapped in gauze (such as an unfolded sterile compress) all across the face and around the eyes. Pat dry with a clean, dry cloth.

BRACING FACIAL FLUID

The ultimate antiaging treatment for dry and sensitive skin, for daily use.

In a small jar with a dropper, add one or two drops of neroli essential oil to two tablespoons of rose hip seed oil. Every night, massage a few drops onto the face and neckline area. This will keep for six months if stored at a steady temperature away from sunlight.

❖ ROSEMARY ❖

Hydrolate, essential oil, flowers, leaves — Origin: Mediterranean region

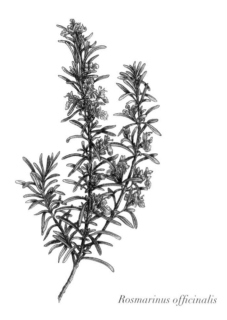

Rosmarinus officinalis

THE TROUBADOURS' HERB

❂

From the Latin *ros marinus*, meaning "sea dew," rosemary is native to the rocky limestone shores of the Mediterranean, where it thrives in a dry climate cooled by the sea spray. According to alternate etymologies, the name derives from the Greek *rhops myrinos* ("aromatic bush"). Used for cooking as well as for treating ailments, rosemary is said to have stimulating, rejuvenating, and disinfecting properties, among others. *Rosmarinus officinalis* is a perennial shrub with pungently aromatic leaves, reputed since antiquity to sharpen the intellect: Greek students wore it in wreaths. "Rosemary is to the spirit what lavender is to the soul," as the saying goes.

TEACHINGS FROM TIME IMMEMORIAL

❂

A symbol of memory, rosemary was ritually burned during funeral ceremonies, for embalming purposes, or as sacred fumigations. The Egyptians would lay a branch in tombs to fortify the spirit of the deceased. Legend has it that its flowers took on the bluish color of the Virgin's mantle after Mary spread it out to dry on the shrub's fragrant branches. Charlemagne decreed that rosemary be cultivated on imperial farms, alongside other medicinal plants with well-established properties. Throughout the Middle Ages, rosemary was ceaselessly celebrated and abundantly used. It was said to possess all manners of benefits, including increasing fertility. Rosemary symbolizes our nascent love for warm days because it grows as early as February. It was first distilled around 1330 for the extraction of its essential oil. In the 16th century, the so-called "Queen of Hungary's Water" was an alcoholic solution of lavender, mint, and rosemary flowers. This miraculous recipe allowed Queen Isabella, who suffered from gout and rheumatism, to recover her health, her youth, and the full measure of her seductive powers past age seventy! The success of this elixir of youth continued to grow until the 17th century. King Louis XIV used it to soothe joint pains in his arm. With its pungent aroma and antiseptic properties, rosemary is also one of the ingredients of the famed "Four Thieves Vinegar" and "*Eau de Cologne*," whose recipe was inherited by perfumer Giovanni Maria Farina in 1736—an alcoholate of rosemary, orange, bitter orange, lemon, bergamot, and neroli. In the 19th century, abbot Sebastian Kneipp recommended the same vivifying recipe, in the form of a rub or a bath, to treat the ailments brought about by aging. Rosemary is also a melliferous plant, whose honey shares its properties. Sailors used this honey as a way of experiencing the plant's benefits during their long crossings.

ON COLLECTING ROSEMARY

◎

Rosemary blooms at the earliest signs of spring and remains in bloom for several months across Southern Europe and around the Mediterranean. It is harvested by hand using a small sickle that cuts off the flowers without damaging them. They are then steam-distilled to produce an essential oil and a hydrolate. One must distinguish between two different types within the *Rosmarinus officinalis* species: *cineoliferum*, the most common one, and *verbenoniferum*, a Corsican variant. The flowers, harvested and left to dry, can be used to make a decoction or an herbal tea.

THE BENEFITS

◎

Rosemary has astringent, purifying, and antiaging properties. The rosmarinic acid it contains in abundance is a potent antioxidant; its terpenes are stimulants, while its cineols and camphor have toning properties. Its essential oil (which should be mixed with a vegetable oil) and its hydrolate are recommended for oily, blemish-prone, mature, or stressed skin, on which they work wonders. Rosemary is also an excellent deodorant and can restore balance to dandruff-prone scalps.

A FEW TWIGS

Nothing is easier than reaping the purifying and astringent benefits of rosemary on the skin: just buy or cut a few twigs and prepare some water.

For a facial treatment, a few branches of rosemary can be thrown into two cups of cold water, brought to a simmer. Maintain the simmer, with the twigs still in, for three minutes; then remove from the heat and allow the rosemary to infuse for seven minutes. Cover your head with a clean, fine-threaded cloth and let your face and mind experience the purifying and reviving effects of rosemary-scented steam.

After cooling, this light rosemary decoction can also be applied as a fortifying hair treatment; use it to rinse the hair after shampooing.

ROSEMARY-BASED RECIPES
from Officine Universelle

THE NEW QUEEN OF HUNGARY'S WATER

This recipe is loosely based on the famed elixir of beauty and youth. A surprising and potent lotion.

In a glass saucepan, simmer (but don't boil!) five handfuls of fresh rosemary flowers in one cup of good champagne and one cup of mineral water for five minutes. The alcohol will partially evaporate; don't keep your nose right above the exhalations. . . . Remove from the heat and allow the preparation to infuse for fifteen minutes. Filter. Once the decoction has cooled down, soak a compress with it and apply it to the face. Refrigerate the rest in a glass jar.

Farewell dull skin and uneven complexions!

LIGHT-FOOTED BATH

Whether you're a hiker or a runner (in high heels during sales season), your feet can't handle it anymore. Plunge them into a relaxing bath, both for their sake and your own. It will also perfume your entire home.

Use 1¾ ounces (fresh) or 1 ounce (dried) each of rosemary, vervain, holy basil, thyme, and borage and two quarts of water to concoct this bath, whose benefits are imparted through transcutaneous exchanges. Rosemary and holy basil, rich in antioxidants, improve stress resistance and stimulate the mind. Vervain fortifies the nervous system. Borage is a fine remedy against premenstrual fatigue and chases melancholy away. Bring the water to a boil and pour it on the herbs in a small tub. Allow to infuse for about thirty minutes before you ease your feet into it, so the water has time to capture the active ingredients and cool down properly. Bathe your feet at length, for fifteen to thirty minutes, reading, for instance, the story of the Bitter Gourd Monk.

Gathering all these ingredients and meditating on the happy asceticism of this Chinese monk is already no small feat. But you can follow it by choosing your preferred oil or cream and patiently massaging the heels and soles of your feet, before launching into a self-pedicure session, using appropriate and well-cleaned instruments.

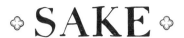

Rice alcohol — Origin: Japan

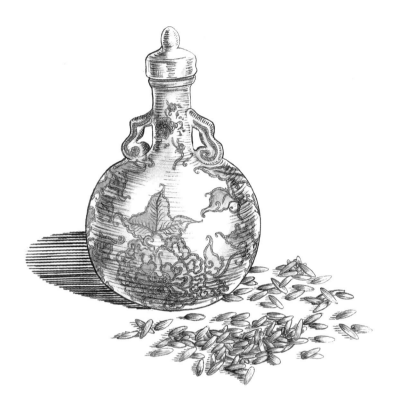

NIHONSHU

○

Although sake – rice alcohol or "wine" – originated in China, it has been present in Japan for millennia, doubtless since the proto-historical period when the cultivation of rice took root. The ancient indigenous religion of the Japanese people, Shinto, keeps its memory alive through the *kami* – supernatural beings and creative forces of nature, ancestral divinities, and spirits – whose benevolent intervention is commonly requested by offering a drink of fermented rice. Historical evidence has shown that sake was used as a ritual alcohol during the imperial feasts of the 4th century AD. It was thus only natural that in the Middle Ages, sake was brewed in temples and sanctuaries, until, as early as the Edo period, sake production took off throughout the archipelago. The grade, notes, and aromas of sake vary depending on water purity, altitude, and temperature, as well as on the brewer's expertise and the extent to which the exterior layer of the sake rice grains is milled – from 20 to 40%, all the way up to 70% for the finest sakes.

> *"Sake for the body,*
> *haiku for the heart."*

SANTOKA

TEACHINGS FROM TIME IMMEMORIAL

Sake brew-masters, or *waza*, are not just esteemed and respected: they are also known for the whiteness of their hands, and the care they bestow upon them. Noticing this quirk, geisha house attendants quickly started caring for their damaged hands with sake, while geishas took to using it for their daily ablutions, so as to enjoy a spotless complexion. At the imperial court, the ladies who dreamed of the luminous, white complexion of the *kami* Amaterasu—goddess of the sun, creator of rice fields and legendary ancestor of the imperial dynasty—did the same. Sake scented with umeboshi (pickled pink plums) became a secret of beauty and youth.

ON PREPARATION

Sake rice is imbued with specific qualities, but it is not edible. The more thoroughly its grain is stone-milled, the more its starchy core is revealed. After being steamed, the mold *Aspergillus oryzae* (a saccharification agent) is sprinkled on the rice. Water is added to this mixture, and alcoholic fermentation works its magic thanks to the yeast *Saccharomyces cerevisiae*.

Sake is made up of 80% water, hence the importance of using water from a pure source.

THE BENEFITS

Sake activates cell turnover, because the sugar obtained from starch fermentation does away with dead cells and brightens the complexion. Its high concentration of vitamin E and oryzanol (an amino acid) means that it makes a fine moisturizer. Ferulic acid (rice yeast) is also a natural antioxidant that protects the skin and preserves its clarity.

A FEW DROPS

It is recommended to apply this surprising facial lotion at night, once all traces of makeup have been removed. Using an untreated cotton pad, apply a small quantity of pure sake (Junmai-grade, preferably) on the face as a lotion. You can also spike your evening bath: one glass for you and three glasses poured into a hot bath for a relaxed body, smooth skin, and a joyful mood!

SAKE-BASED RECIPES
from Officine Universelle

REVIVING, PURIFYING RUBDOWN FOR THE BODY AND NECKLINE AREA

Do you prefer showering to bathing? Develop a taste for a stimulating sake-based rubdown!

Soak a small towel with piping-hot water and wring it out thoroughly, again and again. Pour some gently warmed sake on the damp towel. With no further ado, use it to rub your hands, arms, shoulders, neck, and neckline area, followed by the whole lower body, down to the toes: this treatment activates blood flow, opens up the pores, and gets rid of dead cells and impurities.

DEEP-CLEANING SAKE-BASED FACIAL LOTION

This gentle lotion purifies the complexion and stimulates cell turnover.

In a small jar, mix three tablespoons plus one teaspoon of sake, three tablespoons plus one teaspoon of purified water, and two teaspoons of glycerin. Apply nightly with a cotton pad once all traces of makeup have been removed from the face and neckline area. This mixture can be scented with a drop of lemon balm essential oil.

PURIFYING, ANTI-DANDRUFF LOTION FOR THE SCALP

Many are appalled by the tiny white particles dusting their hair. In order to find a balance, opt for a natural treatment. Apply this treatment once or twice a week during severe bouts of dandruff.

In a small bottle, mix two tablespoons of fine sake, the juice of a large lemon, and a tablespoon of honey. Shake well and keep in the fridge. After shampooing, use it in the final rinse of your hair and scalp. Do not wash it out.

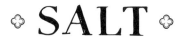 SALT

Salt grains — Origin: World

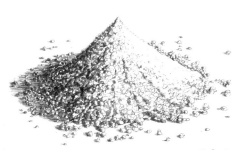

Salarium

WHITE GOLD

Salt, a crystal of sodium chloride, is indispensable to life. Used as a condiment and preservative, it has been harvested in bulk by man since the end of the Neolithic era. Found in the sea and on land, it is stored in the form of slabs or racks, and was used as tender in several ancient cultures. Some Arabic authors mention that salt and gold were given equal value by weight. The "salt roads" have existed since just about forever, and have delineated major lines of communication and trade throughout the world. Men have stretched their ingenuity to collect the precious crystal, whether in coastal salt evaporation ponds or mountain mines. . . . Salt marshes are marvels of technology involving dams, sluice gates, canals, and retention tanks to induce the evaporation of seawater and harvest its salt.

TEACHINGS FROM TIME IMMEMORIAL

Plato called it a substance "beloved of the gods." Offering salt as a gift is a gesture of welcome in several cultures: "friendship is a covenant of salt." Pliny the Elder, in his *Natural History*, described the qualities of salt and its therapeutic virtues at length. In addition to healing crocodile bites and calloused feet, he mentioned, "It is said that teeth never decay nor rot if every morning, before breaking fast, one holds salt under one's tongue until it melts." In the 19th century, a Polish physician, Felix Boczkowski, noticed that salt miners did not suffer from the same respiratory ailments as other miners, and that their health was even much better on average. In 1843, he published a study on the virtues of salt dust and opened the first salt clinic in Krakow. Since the 1960s, halotherapy has been on the rise, offering salt chambers to soothe chronic afflictions of the airways.

ON COLLECTING SALT

Unrefined salt is salt which has undergone no chemical transformation. Raw, often grayish, it is more sensitive to humidity. Salt that was extracted from the earth is called rock salt or halite. It is mined away from air and pollution, in places were ancient seas once evaporated. Salt diamonds are the crude form of rock salt.

196

The salt extracted from salt marshes is richer in taste and in trace elements than its mined counterpart. Fleur de sel is the first layer of these crystals, which is collected on the ground. A more industrial technique consists of forcing evaporation through heating.

THE BENEFITS

Unrefined salt is made up of sodium chloride and a high concentration of mineral salts and trace elements: potassium, magnesium, phosphorus, calcium, iron. It is biologically indispensable to us. It is a tireless ally, which helps improve the body's acid-base balance. Both purifying and cleansing, it soothes irritated skin.

A FEW HANDFULS

Are you already a believer in the virtue of bathing in the sea? Stop limiting the benefits of salt to the warmer months. It is a highly useful ally, which should be brought from the kitchen through to the bathroom. It can very simply be added by the handful to the hot water of full-body or foot baths for relaxation. From the most common to the most exotic, its varieties are as innumerable as its hues and virtues: blue salt from Persia, pink salt from the Andes, black salt from Hawaii or Pakistan. . . .

Handfuls of gray salt
This compacted salt from the bottom of salt ponds is always slightly humid;

it is rich in trace elements and iodine. A little coarse salt ensures quick, efficient exfoliation of damp skin. This scrub effectively alleviates cellulite on affected areas. After use, rinse well with cold water.

Handfuls of Dead Sea salt
This pure unrefined salt has the highest concentration of minerals. It is ideal for soothing atopic skin types and can be used in poultices to heal irritated areas.

Handfuls of pink Himalayan salt
It is extracted from salty rocks found in the mountain range, some 1,640 feet deep. This iodine-free rock salt is used to prepare regenerative and remineralizing baths.

Handfuls of red Hawaiian salt
It owes its hue to a volcanic clay, alaea, which imbues it with beneficial minerals: it is used to make facial scrubs for combination and oily skin types.

Handfuls of Epsom salt
The composition of this bitter salt is very different than that of other salts: it is pure magnesium sulfate. Three handfuls thrown into the bath will relax both body and mind—a most potent treatment for aching muscles.

SALT-BASED RECIPES

from Officine Universelle

BEACH HAIR SPRAY

Keep your mermaid hair after your return to town: make your own "beach spray," a seawater vaporizer.

Dilute one teaspoon of coarse salt in one cup of warm water; add a teaspoon of sesame oil. Whisk in one teaspoon of aloe vera gel. Refrigerate. Shake before applying to the hair.

SUMMER BODY STIMULATING SCRUB

This is the ultimate treatment for the warmer months, combining the hydration of vegetable oils and the energy of salt.

In a bowl, working with your hands, mix three heaping tablespoons of coarse salt and one tablespoon of tamanu oil with one tablespoon of avocado oil. The oil will seep into the salt and start dissolving it. Rub this mixture over the body, focusing on the belly, upper thighs, arms, legs, and ankles. Finish this treatment by showering the whole body with fresh water, being careful not to slip.

HERBAL TOOTHPASTE

This toothpaste, to be used immediately after mixing, will take care of sensitive mouths and freshen the breath.

Mix one teaspoon of fine gray salt with two drops of glycerin, one drop of thyme essential oil, one drop of tea tree essential oil, and one drop of fennel essential oil. Press your damp toothbrush into this mixture. Brush. Rinse. Use within a day and as a balancing treatment once a week.

"Give neither advice nor salt, until you are asked for it."

ENGLISH PROVERB

⊹ SAPOTE ⊹

Kernels, oil — Origin: Mexico

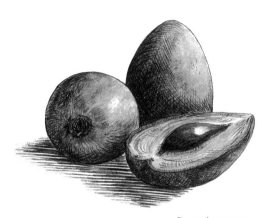

Pouteria sapota

TEACHINGS FROM TIME IMMEMORIAL

◦

The Aztecs prescribed the shell of *tetzonzàpotl* or sapote kernels for sufferers of epilepsy. Roasted and mixed with cocoa, they are an alternative to the more common chocolate. In traditional Cuban medicine, sapote is a classic remedy against gastroenteritis. In the West Indies, the fruit's pulp is also applied as a soothing poultice. In Haiti, Guatemala, and El Salvador, sapote kernel oil is used to ward off baldness.

THE MARMALADE TREE

◦

This tree, native to Central America and also known as mamey, zapote, or lucuma, is from the same family as the argan tree. Its large roundish fruit is not a major export — it doesn't travel well because the brown pulp deteriorates quickly. The flesh of the fruit should be eaten fresh from the tree, with a spoon; it evokes a peculiar mix of sweet potato, avocado, and honey. In Cuba and Haiti, the fruit is enjoyed in sorbets and fruit bars. Planting sapote minimizes soil erosion and provides welcome shade to coffee bushes, which is why these trees are often neighbors.

ON COLLECTING SAPOTE

◦

The fruit contains a kernel which is made up of almost 50% oil. These *zapoyotas* are shelled and the kernels are crushed and sometimes cooked. The oil is extracted by mechanical pressing, then decanted and filtered. It is yellow, with a buttery consistency, and exudes an almond-like scent.

THE BENEFITS

◦

The sapote's spectacular concentration of stearic acid hydrates the skin and hair and protects them too. Oleic acid (omega-9) and palmitic acid are two fatty acids that help moisturize and smooth the skin. The high vitamin A content accelerates cell turnover and evens out freckles and moles, while the vitamin C concentration stimulates microcirculation within the skin and neutralizes free radicals. Nothing in its composition would suggest an ability to encourage hair regrowth, yet in parts of South America, sapote oil is celebrated for just that.

"Use your comb while you have hair on your head."

PROVENÇAL WISDOM

A FEW DROPS

Sapote oil is one of the most esteemed hair fortifiers: if you are losing your hair, or if your mane is battling depression, a weekly scalp massage with sapote oil is an essential part of getting it back into shape. Hurray for curls, frizzy hair, and triumphant afros! A few drops of sapote oil, warmed between your palms and applied to damp hair, will enable you to tame and maintain it. If the oil has solidified, run some warm water over it.

SAPOTE-BASED RECIPES
from Officine Universelle

CARIBBEAN STRONG HAIR MASK
If you can't live on the beach, prepare this fortifying mask for yourself instead.

Using a small bamboo whisk, carefully mix two tablespoons of sapote oil, one organic egg yolk, and one tablespoon of rum in a bowl. Apply this as a poultice on washed, damp hair and leave on for thirty minutes. Rinse off with a second gentle shampoo. Wring out your hair and allow it to air-dry instead of rubbing and drying it using a towel.

❖ SEA BUCKTHORN ❖

Oil (berries) — Origin: Eurasia

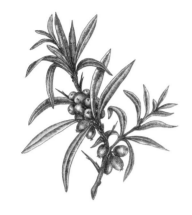

Hippophae rhamnoides

THE SIBERIAN PINEAPPLE

○

Hippophae rhamnoides, a diminutive shrub with silver-green foliage, thrives on rocky terrain, whether mountainous or coastal. This heliophilous variety colonizes stony ground and dunes, basking in the sun and thus preventing the terrible erosion of very dry soil. In summer, the shrub's spiny branches adorn themselves with small yellow and orange fruits. The sea buckthorn has only been intensively cultivated for its fruit since the 1950s. China has the world's largest sea buckthorn orchards.

TEACHINGS FROM TIME IMMEMORIAL

○

Legend has it that the branches and fruit of the sea buckthorn were the favorite food of Pegasus, the divine winged horse of Greek mythology. Pliny the Elder described the sea buckthorn and a related species in his *Natural History*: "These two plants have great properties for horses, which is why they were named *hippophae*." The branches and fruit of the plant, which is often used for horse feed, were reputed to impart shine to the steeds' coats, hence its pleasant Latin name, which means "glossy horse." In Mongolia, the shrub grows in the wild and nomads used to turn it into soups and juice. The Mongol emperor Genghis Khan himself ate it as a fortifier. The Russians were among the first to take an interest in its properties and its unbelievable vitamin C content, which is thirty times that of an orange. They included it in the diet of the first Russian astronauts, who also applied its oil to shield themselves from cosmic radiation. In present-day China, more than two hundred different foodstuffs are based on sea buckthorn.

ON COLLECTING SEA BUCKTHORN

○

The spines of the sea buckthorn complicate the harvest, and the fruit is picked after the onset of the first nighttime frosts, which cause the branches to shed their leaves. Its berries are highly sensitive to oxidation and must be either frozen or pressed immediately. The red-tinted oil, with its fruity and peppery scent, can be extracted from the seeds when the fruit is first pressed, or from the pomace that is left following this first pressing. The oil derived from the first pressing is more precious than that which is obtained by pressing the pomace.

THE BENEFITS

Sea buckthorn oil has a remarkable concentration of fatty acids and vitamins. Its vitamin E content is astonishing: it neutralizes the action of free radicals and helps the skin fight external aggressions. The oil is very rich in carotenoids (or pro-vitamin A); it minimizes the devastating effects of exposure to the sun's rays and soothes irritated skin.

A FEW DROPS

This plant, which is fond of extreme climates, yields an oil that protects the skin from sun, wind, and cold. A few drops of sea buckthorn oil will work wonders after a long day on snowy slopes, while for city dwellers, sea buckthorn oil is beneficial for skin that is irritated or otherwise affected by pollution and the other hassles of modern life. For the most sensitive skin types, which have become intolerant or have overindulged in the sun, daily use is soothing and potent. A few drops mixed with an organic hydrating body milk will extend the benefits of sea buckthorn to the entire body and enable a safe passage through summer.

SEA BUCKTHORN–BASED RECIPES

from Officine Universelle

ANTI-REDNESS YOUTH SERUM

Your skin bruises easily and, despite your repeated efforts, is prone to redness. This serum provides consummate care and ensures a return to normalcy.

In a small jar with a dropper, mix one part sea buckthorn oil, one part raspberry seed oil, and one part pomegranate oil. Apply to thoroughly clean skin, after removing all traces of makeup, as often as required, in the morning and at night.

SUBSOLAR OIL

La dolce vita – a body and facial oil for lounging on the beach or at a terrace bar.

Fill a small jar with a dropper with one part sea buckthorn oil and one part wheat bran oil, and add three drops of true lavender essential oil. Hurray for the summery pleasure of a radiant tan on pretty skin!

❖ SEAWEEDS ❖

Whole plant — Origin: Asia

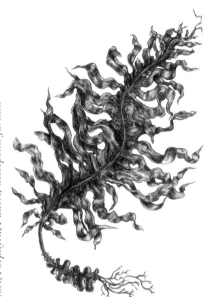

Wakame, Undaria pinnatifida, Kombu, Saccharina japonica, Nori, Porphyra, Funori, Gloiopeltis furcata

TAKE TO THE SEA

◦

Seaweeds make up a highly heterogeneous group of about one hundred freshwater and saltwater plants. Their size varies from a few millimeters to thirty or more feet. They can be as modest as dull grass or, on the contrary as sumptuous and flamboyant as fantastical hairdos; they cover the full range of possible hues and shapes, and can be divided into three large groups: green, red, and brown. Cultivating the marine species of seaweeds only started in the early 20th century. Nowadays, the bulk of seaweed production comes from Asia, where brown varieties predominate.

TEACHINGS FROM TIME IMMEMORIAL

◦

The mythological Chinese emperor of "ox-head" fame, Shennong, is said to have detailed the therapeutic benefits of seaweeds in his phytotherapy treatise, *Shennong bencaojing*. Since the dawn of time, these submerged plants have been praised for their diuretic, fortifying, tonifying, and regenerative action. In Asia, seaweeds are a symbol of health and well-being; the best ones were reserved for dignitaries and nobles. In 701, the Japanese empire decreed that the date of February 6 in its calendar would from then on be known as the annual seaweed day. Nori and arame, two of the archipelago's reigning seaweeds, were mentioned in the list of the most precious foods that could be put before the emperor. In 931, a Chinese-Japanese dictionary listed twenty-one species of edible seaweeds, offering advice on their proper preparation. A choice food in numerous coastal regions around the world, seaweeds remained an untapped resource in Europe and North America for a long time: they were used as cattle feed and people would only eat them in times of famine. In the 16th century, William Turner, the father of English botany, called them "the useful grasses." In the 13th century, the Salerno School noted the beneficial effects of dried seaweeds and of seaweed ashes to prevent the development

> *"Seaweeds are a delicacy, to be offered to the most honorable guests."*

SZE TEU

of goiter. It wasn't until the 19th century with the rise of thalassotherapy that the West belatedly recognized the virtues of the marine environment and of the seaweeds that thrive there. In Flanders, the story goes that before his departure overseas, a fisherman had given his fiancée a splendid marine grass, finely cut. As the young man's absence was weighing on her heart, the girl set about replicating the wonderful seaweed with lace, promising that should the young sailor return safe and sound from those distant lands, she would forgo the marriage and devote herself to worshiping the Virgin Mary. Once her handiwork was complete, her fiancé returned. On the day her beloved came back, the girl brought her wonderful handiwork before Mary, spreading it on the altar and crying all the way. A miracle occurred and these liberating words appeared on the holy table: "I free you from your vow." Soon marrying her beloved, she became famous for her lacework, which became highly prized throughout the land.

ON COLLECTING ALGAE

Algaculture is now in constant development: close to 90% of seaweed on sale is the product of cultivation. This often involves the immersion of frames, which the plants easily latch on to, into the sea or in freshwater. Nori is cultivated in Japan in nets that are suspended in shallow waters. At low tide, the seaweeds are exposed to the air. They are harvested during the winter, thoroughly rinsed with seawater, cut into little pieces and left to dry on racks, and finally compressed into thin, sheet-like layers that are easy to cook. Kombu is left to dry in the sun, then forgotten in a cellar for two years! Wakame leaves are separated from the stem and then dehydrated in dry heat or preserved in salt.

A FEW LEAVES

The preparing of seaweed-based beauty treatments requires a taste for experimentation, sea legs, and a seaworthy nose! Their ability to eliminate toxins and their stimulating properties are beyond compare. One can simply add a pinch of powdered seaweed to a neutral organic shampoo or a simple clay mask. For an instant radiance boost, nothing is easier than soaking a few wakame leaves in mineral water for a few minutes and then applying them to the face to absorb their benefits. Wait for ten to fifteen minutes before removing them, then run a rose water-soaked cotton pad over the face, to achieve in minutes what would take a whole weekend at the beach. . . .

SEAWEED-BASED RECIPES

from Officine Universelle

BEAUTIFUL SHORELINE RINSE

Never again limit seaweeds to that all-too-rare week of thalassotherapy.

Pour a bowl of boiling mineral water onto two pieces of dried kombu in a porcelain bowl (metal demineralizes). Cover with a small dish and allow to infuse for thirty minutes before removing the seaweed, which you can later use for cooking. After shampooing, rinse your hair with this infused water, then with cold water.

PURPLE SEAWEED FORTIFYING SHAMPOO

If nothing is too beautiful or exotic for your hair, then this marine shampoo was made for you!

Drop a handful of funori seaweed into a glass saucepan, remove from the heat immediately after it starts boiling, cover, and allow to cool down. Filter the liquid through a cloth, applying heavy pressure to the seaweed. Apply this rosy gel to the whole hair for about ten minutes, then rinse several times with clear water, and follow by rinsing with water spiked with cider vinegar.

DEEP-SEA BATH

Indulge in this shock treatment to improve your figure and combat fatigue! Perform as a weekly cure in winter, or once a month for year-round maintenance.

First, take a tepid shower and gently exfoliate the body with coarse salt. Use unsalted food-grade seaweeds: kombu, wakame, funori. Fill a large cotton bag with said seaweeds and allow to infuse for twenty minutes in a very hot bath. Once it has cooled down a bit, step into the bath and remain for about twenty minutes. Once out of the bath, don a warm, dry bathrobe and lie down for fifteen minutes under a blanket, with your head and feet propped up.

❖ SESAME ❖

Oil (seeds) — Origin: India

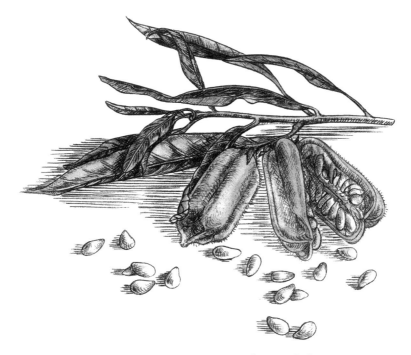

Sesamum indicum

"OPEN SESAME"

T his plant from the Lamiaceae family is a Southern belle: India and Africa are the world's foremost producers. Sesame doesn't spark interest because of its trumpet-shaped flowers, which can be pink or white depending on altitude, but rather for the myriad little seeds it holds in its pods. When fully matured, these pods open up suddenly, as a lock might . . ..

TEACHINGS FROM TIME IMMEMORIAL

The Latin name comes from the Akkadian and Phoenician languages. In China, it is called *moa*, *goma* in Japan, *tila* in Sanskrit. According to Herodotus, the Greek historian, the Babylonians were the earliest consumers of sesame oil. Assyrian mythology says that the gods got drunk on sesame wine just before they created the world. In the Indus Valley, in Harappa, excavations have unearthed six-thousand-year-old leftovers of roasted sesame. In India, according to the *Brahma Purana*, the god of death, Yama, created sesame, which became a symbol of life and immortality. In 1520, the Portuguese traveler Domingo Paes was staying at the court of the Vijayanagara Empire, in Southern India. He reported the sovereign's morning routine: "Each day before dawn, the King drinks a measure of sesame oil and anoints his body with it. He covers his waist with a piece of cloth, grabs a very heavy weight with one hand, and then takes his saber in the other hand and trains until he has sweated all the oil out." Ayurveda—the Indian holistic philosophy and medicine, or "science of life"—has cemented the reputation of sesame oil as beneficial for healing aching joints as well as purifying and freeing the mind: in the latter case it is poured, warm, in a continuous flow over the forehead and massaged in. Traditional Chinese medicine recommends application of sesame oil to soothe minor burns, and includes it in the diet of breastfeeding mothers. In Buddhist practice, throwing sesame seeds into a fire and breathing in the smoke helps the body heal. Sesame, which is considered medicinal there, is thus omnipresent in the Mediterranean culinary heritage: from tahini to halva, through the Berber *zamita* or *zmeta*. The seeds can be sprinkled on bread before it's baked to boost its flavor. Today, the seed is a staple of macrobiotic diets.

ON COLLECTING SESAME

The stems of the plant are hand-cut before maturity because the seed-filled pods are fragile. Once they're tied into sheaves, the stems are shaken over sheets to collect the tiny seeds that fall from the opened pods. Elongated and somewhat flat, the seeds can be black, red, golden, or white. The darkest come from Asia (India, China, or Japan), the palest from the Middle East and the West. Their oil content oscillates between 50 and 70%. For cosmetic uses, the seeds must not be roasted before they are cold-pressed. The oil's sesame scent is mild, and its texture enables ready absorption.

THE BENEFITS

Because sesame oil is rich in natural antioxidants (sesamoline, lecithin, and vitamin E), it helps the cells fight oxidative stress. Its linoleic acid (omega-6) concentration protects the skin from outside aggressions and efficiently prevents it from drying. Oleic acid (omega-9) nourishes it, helps with the scarification of minor scrapes, and soothes pruritus.

A FEW DROPS

Pure sesame oil, thanks to its fine texture and mild scent, is ideal for body massages or soothing irritated scalps. Beware: sesame is a common allergen—before anointing your body or hair with it, massage a drop on the inside of your wrist and wait to see if an allergic reaction occurs.

SESAME-BASED RECIPES
from Officine Universelle

PURIFYING, MAKEUP-REMOVING OIL

Down with preconceived notions! Combination skin can greatly benefit from select vegetable oils. This potent balancing and purifying trio should be resorted to on a daily basis.

In a small jar, mix one part sesame oil, one part jojoba oil, and one part nigella oil. Apply on a damp cotton pad and run over the face to clean it.

GANDOUSH

Merely brushing your teeth will not guarantee oral hygiene! Complete daily cleansing with this Indian recipe.

Upon waking up, on an empty stomach, take 2½ teaspoons of sesame oil and run it around your mouth for a few minutes, from side to side, over your gums and palate. Some purists recommend doing this for at least twenty minutes. . . . Then spit it out and rinse your mouth with warm water. Do this every day, or when detoxing.

HANANOTSUYU, OR FLOWER DEW

Invented in the 17th century, this remedy is used to fight unsightly blemishes and bring radiance to the face. It is also used as a nourishing treatment for the hair.

Fill a small jar three-quarters of the way with virgin sesame oil, then immerse a small piece of sandalwood and three organic cloves in the oil. Allow to macerate for about ten days, regularly shaking the contents. Filter and repeat: perform a second maceration, using the same quantities, and filter again. Apply to your freshly cleansed face at night, right before bed. This can also be used as a conditioner on well-rinsed hair: smooth the hair with a comb dipped into some hot water and spiked with five drops of sesame oil.

EGYPTIAN OIL

If your loved ones are lucky enough to enjoy your talents as a masseuse, Egyptian oil helps your hands unknot tensions more efficiently.

Finely grate 1.4 ounces of fresh organic ginger over a very fine cloth. Press to extract the juice and add it to three tablespoons of sesame oil, along with half a teaspoon of organic lemon juice. Keep in a small jar with a dropper. Shake well before embarking on a massage.

ST. JOHN'S WORT

Macerate (flowers) — Origin: Europe

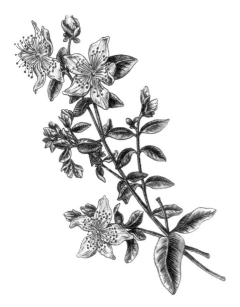

Hypericum perforatum

DEVIL'S SCOURGE

With their deep, radiant yellow hue, the corollas of these flowers adorn the sides of country lanes and dot clearings, which they perfume with an intoxicating scent. The flowers and stems of this variant, sometimes known as "Perforate St. John's wort" ("perforate" because the leaves are punctured by tiny openings), contain high concentrations of a precious substance: hypericin, a potent, deep-red anti-inflammatory active ingredient, whose name was reportedly inspired by Hyperion, the Titan of Greek mythology. Throughout the European countryside, it has always been said that St. John's wort repelled witches and chased the devil away. . . . Its (more rational) medicinal and cosmetic properties are now officially recognized.

TEACHINGS FROM TIME IMMEMORIAL

Legendary princess Nausicaa, whose beauty is lauded by Ulysses in *The Odyssey*, reportedly used St. John's wort to care for her face and body. In antiquity, physicians favored St. John's wort ointments and unguents to heal wounds and burns. Such remedies can be found in the works of the Roman naturalist Pliny the Elder, and of the Greek physician and botanist Pedanius Dioscorides. Above all, it is one of the constituents of the famed theriac—the remedy and antidote crafted by Andromachus, personal physician to the Roman emperor Nero. Reworked and improved by apothecaries over the centuries, this panacea, reputedly a cureall, was only removed from the codex in the late 19th century. In the 16th century, the *eau d'arquebusade*, an officinal tincture of St. John's wort prepared by monks, healed the wounds of arquebus-wielding soldiers—hence its name. In the 18th century, St. John's wort could be found in the formula of the famed "Commander's Balm," a mixture said to be antiseptic. The flowers of this sacred plant, used in St. John's Day celebrations, were plucked before daybreak, with a pure heart (that's the hard part!) and bare feet, walking backwards. St. John's wort is a plant with a magical, sunny aura, which symbolizes victory over the forces of darkness and evil. Thus, it was customary to sleep with St. John's wort under one's pillow as a protection against death. . . . Incidentally, in 1525, Paracelsus noted its action against "the evil spells that push men into despair": he was doubtlessly predicting its natural potency against despondency (or depression in modern terms), a property that is now well established.

ON COLLECTING ST. JOHN'S WORT

❁

Harvested immediately after blooming from May through September, the flowers and half the stems are put out to dry. For cosmetic uses, the active ingredients are captured by macerating the fresh flowers for several weeks in a neutral natural oil, which then takes on a beautiful yellow tint. It is recommended not to apply St. John's wort macerate prior to sun exposure, for hypericin makes the skin more photosensitive.

THE BENEFITS

❁

Hyperforin naturally fosters the scarification process and helps reduce inflammation. In this respect, it is supported by hypericin, which has potent anti-inflammatory properties. Its high tannin concentration gives it excellent astringency, while its flavonoids are efficient antioxidants, which help fight the signs of aging.

A FEW DROPS

Everyone should keep a small vial of St. John's wort macerate in their vanity case. Its application can be extremely potent in combating mild burns and sunburn. It is an especially stalwart ally of intolerant and reactive skin types. To be applied at night only, due to its tendency to increase photosensitivity. Among other emergency applications, it can help reduce muscle stiffness after sport: drink generous amounts of Vichy water and massage St. John's wort macerate into your aching muscles. St John's wort is also said to increase one's libido. . . .

ST. JOHN'S WORT–BASED RECIPES

from Officine Universelle

YOUR OWN MACERATE

You can always buy it from a store, but nothing beats the pleasure of doing things yourself, and of choosing the precious oil which is to harvest the wonderful virtues of St. John's wort.

Select a small jar with a wide opening. Fill halfway with dried flowers of St. John's wort and cover with jojoba oil. Seal the jar and allow to macerate for four weeks, regularly turning the jar upside down. Filter through a piece of cotton gauze (such as a cheesecloth), pressing down on the flowers so as not to waste any macerate, then pour the oil into a sterilized airtight container.

This macerate has numerous uses: healing a newborn's cradle cap, relieving aching muscles and joints after excessive exercise, soothing irritated skin after sunburn — or a regular burn.

WINTER BLUES MASSAGE OIL

In the depths of winter, under a gray, gray sky, the five p.m. nightfall can seriously impact your morale: put St. John's wort's solar flower power to use!

In a three-ounce jar with a dropper, mix one part St. John's wort macerate with one part hydrating and emollient jojoba oil; then add five drops of irritation-fighting Roman chamomile essential oil and ten drops of anti-infectious marjoram oil. At bedtime, massage a few drops of this comforting mixture onto the whole body.

PHAEACIA FACIAL OIL

Does your skin take offense to just about anything? From one redness to the next inflammation, is there nothing you'll be spared? Enough! Apply this fluid made of beneficial oils at bedtime every night for a month, to recover some peace and quiet.

In a two-ounce jar with a dropper, mix one part St. John's wort macerate, which helps with scarification, and one part antiaging, brightening rose hip seed oil, adding five drops of astringent and purifying rosemary essential oil and three drops of anti-inflammatory true lavender essential oil. Apply just before bedtime, after removing all traces of makeup.

✤ SWEET ALMOND ✤

Oil (kernel) — Origin: Mediterranean basin

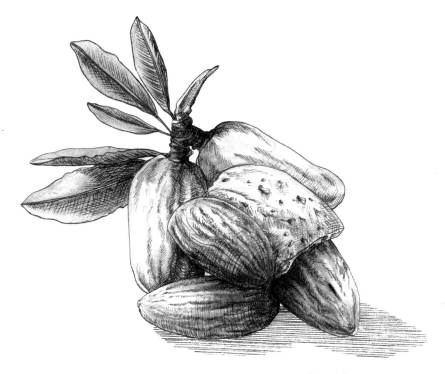

Prunus amygdalus dulcis

THE MIRACLE OF MANDORLE

Originally, the wild almond tree, known since time immemorial from the Pamir to the Aegean Sea, only yielded tiny, very bitter kernels. . . . It is impossible to know when its cultivation started through the progressive selection of sweeter-tasting, more highly prized fruit. It was reportedly introduced by the Greeks, and later spread through the Mediterranean basin along with the Roman expansion, from Italy on to Spain and Southern France. The Romans called the fruit of the sweet almond tree "the Greek nut." The almond is covered by a velvety skin, resembling a thin, very pale green fuzz; this covers a hard shell which conceals the kernel. This oily dried fruit comes in more than fifty varieties, such as the Italian "Avola," the Tunisian "Sfax," the Spanish "Marcona," and the French "Princesse." Nowadays, California has become the almond tree's new homeland, producing more than half the global harvest. Local beekeepers have had to rent beehives to keep up with the intensive pollination. The almond, falling victim to the worldwide enthusiasm it has elicited, may well become a precious commodity. . . .

TEACHINGS FROM TIME IMMEMORIAL

The cosmetic use of sweet almond has been documented for millennia. For relaxing massages, Egyptian ladies from the Late Period used to coat their bodies with an ointment made from sweet almond, honey, and cinnamon. . . . For the Greeks, it symbolized the faith and love incarnated by Phyllis, who died when she could no longer bear waiting for her lover's return and was turned into an almond tree by the goddess Hera, out of pity. The almond represents fertility, much like its flowers blooming on the bare branches of the tree before the leaves come out. Legend even has it that a young virgin sleeping under an almond tree could wake up and find herself pregnant. The almond was also a symbol of happiness and plenty for the Romans, who used to throw handfuls of them on newlyweds to bring them good luck. These intertwined beliefs explain why, in many countries, the sugared almond is an indispensable gift at weddings, baptisms, and the like. *These white flowers that will bring almonds to wed girls and boys*, as a poem from the Provence region puts it. In the 12th century, Hildegarde de Bingen recommended the consumption of almonds to revive the brain's vigor and the complexion's radiance. Another tale has it that in Portugal, when the Algarve was ruled by the Moors, an Arabic prince fell for a princess from the north with blond hair and blue eyes. They got married, and there was much rejoicing, but over time, the princess fell into melancholy: her nostalgia for the snow-covered fields of her homeland was growing. Her husband decreed that almond trees be planted throughout the Algarve. In the springtime, he invited the princess to behold the view from atop the ramparts: the countryside, filled with almond flowers, appeared thoroughly white to her eyes, as if covered in snow. Her sadness vanished forever.

ON COLLECTING SWEET ALMOND OIL

The almonds harvested during the year are shelled, and each kernel is steam-processed to remove its seedcoat. Once they are clean, they are cold-pressed and filtered. Four and a half pounds of almonds will yield one quart of oil. Good sweet almond oil is faintly tinted, almost transparent; it must not look cloudy, and should exude a very light, never pungent aroma.

THE BENEFITS

Sweet almond oil has universal appeal—it is a family-friendly treatment that will suit children and babies splendidly. Its high concentration of oleic acid (omega-9) and vitamin E softens and soothes the skin: it alleviates minor itches and common inflammations. Vitamins B1, B2, and B6, which it contains naturally, stimulate the synthesis of keratin, thus enriching the hair and the nails. However, beware: it is recommended that people with nut allergies refrain from using it.

"Kisses are like almonds."

JUST A FEW DROPS

Sweet almond oil is a quintessential beauty remedy. The old as well as the young will find that the benefits and the ease of use justify its presence in any bathroom. Day in, day out, it is a moisturizer that will heal a variety of minor skin issues. A few drops will pacify the irritated bottoms of infants, and alleviate chapped and dry skin for the whole family.

SWEET ALMOND OIL–BASED RECIPES

from Officine Universelle

GENTLE EXFOLIANT FOR THE FACE AND LIPS

After a few days of joyful excess or worrisome stress, this will bring a new radiance to your complexion.

Soak five shelled almonds (with their seedcoats removed) for several hours. Crush to a powder using a mortar and pestle, then mix with one tablespoon of honey and one tablespoon of whole milk. Mix thoroughly using a bamboo whisk and leave on the face for ten minutes. Then, making small circular motions, massage this paste like a scrub on the uneven or dry areas of the face, and do so even more gently on the lips. Carefully rinse and pat dry. There you are, your fresh complexion is back!

FORTIFYING OIL FOR THE HAIR AND SCALP

This Sunday treatment must be applied several weeks in a row — early in the season, it will stimulate hair growth and balance the scalp's production of sebum.

Mix one tablespoon of sweet almond oil, one tablespoon of castor seed oil, and one teaspoon of tamanu oil. Massage into your scalp and finish by running your fingers along the lengths of your hair. Keep your hair warm for thirty minutes (or overnight . . .) under a dry, fine towel, a turban, or a scarf. A soothing session with your hair is a great way to start your week.

✤ TAMANU ✤

Kernel, oil — Origin: Oceania, Polynesia, and Africa

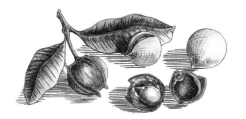

Calophyllum inophyllum

THE PACIFIC TREE

○

Calophyllum inophyllum is a large tree from the Clusiaceae family with opulently green foliage, native to the coasts of East Africa, Southern India, and Australia. After the hundreds of clusters of flowers it carries have bloomed, its branches are covered in round, smooth, pea-green fruit, or drupes. Inside each of these, a kernel contains all the benefits of the tamanu, a sacred tree in Polynesia.

TEACHINGS FROM TIME IMMEMORIAL

○

Also known as the "Alexandrian laurel," the tamanu tree is planted within Polynesian places of worship, because of the traditional belief that gods like to come and rest in its cool shade. The tree's ritual use was highly codified: its wood, for example, was used for the creation of *tiki* — anthropomorphic statues, statuettes or amulets. In the traditional pharmacopeia, it is considered a *ra'au*

tahiti — a medicine and a panacea. The leaves help cure skin conditions, while the blossoms (along with Tiaré flowers) are a constituent part of *monoï*. The juice from its fruit is prescribed as a cure for headaches, and Tahitian mothers have always cared for their babies by massaging them with tamanu oil. Western science is still investigating and uncovering the oil's numerous and mysterious powers.

PREPARATION

○

Once the ripe drupes have been harvested, the nuts are separated from the pulp and laid out to dry in the sun for several weeks. This drying treatment causes the oil concentration to rise. The nuts are then cold-pressed, releasing a yellow-green substance with an almost spicy scent. Those who have a taste for it find this aroma incomparably delicious.

THE BENEFITS

○

Tamanu oil has a high concentration of linoleic acid—an omega-6—which acts as a protective agent for the skin, and vitamin E, which skillfully prevents cell oxidation. It's exceptionally rich in oleic acid—omega-9—and in aminophylline, calaustraline, and inophyllolide, which help the scarring process of skin and heal small flesh wounds. As for the lauric acid, it fights inflammations and decongests the skin, while polyphenols enhance microcirculation.

A FEW DROPS

This efficacious oil is imbued with so many benefits that it could become an everyday treatment and an essential addition to any beauty kit. Because of its potency, try one drop on the inside of your arm prior to use.

Gently dabbed under the eyes, it alleviates dark rings, bags and signs of fatigue; applied topically, it treats irritations as well as the skin's driest areas; used as an ointment on the scalp it soothes irritations, and balances and reinforces the hair.

TAMANU-BASED RECIPES
from Officine Universelle

ANTI–STRETCH MARK SERUM

Rub, scrub . . . find the method that works best for you to effect deep body exfoliation once a week! Combined with the nightly application of this fluid, this will improve the appearance of your skin.

In an opaque large jar with a dropper, carefully mix 40% tamanu oil, 30% baobab seed oil, and 30% grapeseed oil—along with a few drops of *Helichrysum italicum* (aka "Immortal") essential oil, for its properties and for comfort's sake.

Stretch marks are a common and regrettable nuisance, but applying a regular treatment will make them look much more presentable.

ANTI-ROSACEA FACIAL OIL

Are you infuriated by your skin's sensitivity to changes in the weather? Keep in mind that the sun is your worst enemy. Are you waging war on these tiny red marks? Is your skin often intolerant? You must limit the inflammation and choose a natural and beneficial ritual.

In an opaque large jar with a dropper, carefully mix 20% tamanu oil, 10% St. John's wort oil, and 70% black currant oil.

Opt for regular, preventative use.

❖ TEA ❖

Leaves, buds — Origin: Asia

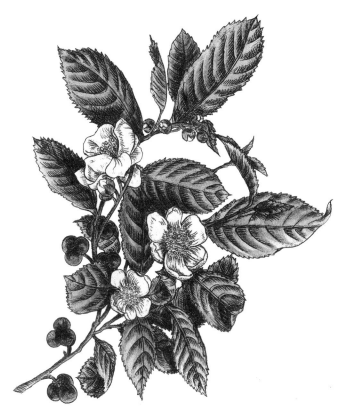

Camellia sinensis or *Thea sinensis*

LEAF BY LEAF

In the wild, depending on the variety, this evergreen shrub can reach heights of between sixteen and fifty feet. Like many tropical species, *Camellia sinensis* alternates between periods of intense growth and periods of rest. Only the vegetative part of the plant—the bud and the two leaves that are attached to it—is harvested. When it comes to growing tea, the name of the game is to avoid the beautiful, white, and fragrant blossoming of the tree, so as to maintain it in a permanent state of vegetative growth. Cultivating it requires a warm, even climate: it thrives more readily in elevated equatorial regions. One tea leaf contains more caffeine than a coffee bean. Nowadays, tea is the most widely consumed drink in the world, after water.

TEACHINGS FROM TIME IMMEMORIAL

○

A 6th-century legend says that a Hindu monk, Bodhidharma, who had come to China to preach the Chan school of Buddhism, had vowed not to sleep for nine years. Yet after a few years, he fell asleep at the foot of a tree. Angry with himself, he cut off his eyelids and buried them. At this exact spot, a plant named *tch'a*, whose leaves looked like eyelids, took root. Consuming it enabled him to stay awake. . . . China prides itself on owning the world's oldest tea trees. It is said that tea originates from Xishuangbanna, a region in Yunnan Province, where a famed tea tree named *Bada* is reportedly 1,700 years old. Drinking tea as an infusion, which in China goes back to the 8th century BC, is elaborated upon in the *Shijing*, the *Book of Songs*. Tea clarifies the spirit, eases digestion, and neutralizes toxins, according to Chinese medicine. In Japan, where beauty is tackled holistically—with an emphasis on the outside appearance reflecting inner well-being—the "Way of Tea" is the name of a way of being, an aesthetic, almost an art, connected to the tea ceremony. Tea was introduced in Europe by the Portuguese in the 16th century. It became popular a century later through its trade by the French East India Company.

ON COLLECTING TEA

○

Tea cultivation is a perennial affair: the leaves are plucked periodically throughout the year, at varying intervals depending on the region and season.

In Darjeeling, India, one of the world's most celebrated tea-growing regions, the leaves are harvested more than forty times a year. The first harvest of the new year, after winter has allowed the leaves to get highly concentrated in essential oils, is the most highly prized. The harvest is performed manually, often with no other tool than the tea picker's fingers. In order to keep the tea green, natural oxidation is arrested through quick heat-drying. In Japan, the leaves are steamed, which is the surest way to preserve their vitamins. For black tea, the leaves are left to wilt for about twenty hours, and are then rolled to hasten oxidation. Once the proper level of oxidation has been reached, the leaves are exposed to an elevated temperature so as to stop the process.

THE BENEFITS

○

With its high concentration of polyphenols, including highly effective epigallocatechin gallate (EGCG), green tea is a potent antioxidant. The presence of tannins further enhances this action. Its high caffeine content makes it an efficient booster in slimming treatments.

A FEW PINCHES

Prepare the most effective of radiance-boosting treatments: a teaspoon of powdered green tea (matcha), emulsified in your preferred vegetable oil (wheat germ is ideal for lifeless complexions . . .). Compresses soaked with warm tea will soothe and decongest weary eyes.

TEA-BASED RECIPES

from Officine universelle

━━◆━━

MIZUDASHI LOTION

Why make anything more complicated than it has to be? Combine the pleasures and the vitamin-rich virtues of iced green tea – both as a drink and a lotion.

Preserve the properties of green tea thanks to the cold extraction of a handful of sencha tea leaves in two cups of mineral water. Allow to infuse in the fridge for at least two hours. Drink a glass of this iced tea while running a tea-soaked cotton pad over your face.

A refreshing radiance booster, to be enjoyed as often as is necessary during heat waves.

GREEN TEA BATH SALT

For those who swear by bathing in the morning, this highly invigorating bath salt will make it easier to face the day.

Into a glass or ceramic bowl, pour a level tablespoon of powdered green tea, known as "matcha," and three level tablespoons of unrefined coarse sea salt, and mix thoroughly after adding three drops of the natural oil of your choice. Pour this mixture under the stream of hot water, allow to melt and infuse for three minutes, stirring the water, then step into the tub.

GO GREEN

In the privacy of your bathroom, transform yourself into a little green man under this preventive mask, which alleviates the noxious effects of "oxidative stress" – whether from the weather, the office environment, or pollution peaks.

In a glass or ceramic bowl, mix 2½ teaspoons of powdered green tea (matcha), one tablespoon of superfine Pascalite clay, and one tablespoon of lemon balm hydrolate. Gently apply to the face. Leave on for about ten minutes, then rinse with fresh water.

SLIMMING BODY SCRUB

No miracle here: only regular exfoliation and massage of the most sensitive areas will improve the skin's appearance. And to that end, tea is a stalwart ally!

In a glass or ceramic bowl, mix one tablespoon of green tea, one teaspoon of organic brown sugar, and one tablespoon of daisy macerate. Rub this mixture over the body, focusing on the belly, upper thighs, arms, legs, and ankles. Finish this treatment by showering the whole body with fresh water, being careful not to slip.

❖ TEA TREE ❖

Essential oil (leaves) — Origin: Australia

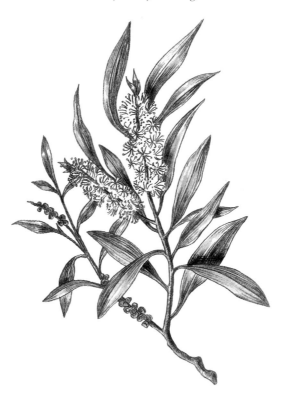

Melaleuca alternifolia

BUSH MEDICINE

◉

Melaleuca alternifolia is a "sempervirens" tree, an evergreen whose leaves exude a characteristic smell. Although confusingly known as the "tea tree," it has nothing in common with the tea plant *Camellia sinensis*. The tree thrives on the marshy soils of New South Wales and Queensland, Australia, where it multiplies easily thanks to its suckers. This vigorous and generous species is ripe for its first harvest after a year and a half of growth.

TEACHINGS FROM TIME IMMEMORIAL

◉

This tree is the green gold of indigenous Australians. The Bundjalung people were its first documented users: they would crush its leaves to a powder or a paste, which featured in remedies against skin irritations and wounds. Dark water lakes, lined with tea trees, were sacred places where women would go to give birth. Nowadays, it is still recommended to swim in such places to benefit from the virtues of this peculiar freshwater. Feeling nostalgic for his customary cup of tea, the famed explorer James Cook named the plant "tea tree" after using its leaves in an infusion as a substitute for actual tea. He mentions it in the diary of his second expedition in 1777. The Australian scientist A. R. Penford was the first to study the plant's properties. His conclusions, published in 1925, were stupefying: the antiseptic action of *Melaleuca* is thirteen times more efficient than that of phenic acid, which is used for the same reasons. A national craze was born and has endured ever since: during the Second World War, every Australian soldier received a small vial of tea tree oil to furnish his emergency kit.

ON PREPARING TEA TREE OIL

Until the 1980s, harvesting tea tree leaves and twigs meant picking them in the wild, which was rather exhausting work. Nowadays, the tree is cultivated in plantations. Cutting it requires a certain amount of know-how, since the leaves' oil reserve can be damaged by an imprecise motion or treatment. The tree's geographic origin is significant, since its composition varies greatly from one region to the next. The leaves and twigs are distilled in vaporization chambers. Tea tree essential oil is colorless, sometimes with a very pale yellow tint, with a highly distinctive and sustained woody and camphorous scent.

THE BENEFITS

Tea tree essential oil is one of the greatest and most effective natural antiseptics. The monoterpenols it contains, especially terpinen-4-ol, are impressive, wide-ranging anti-infectious agents that are well tolerated by the skin. Monoterpenes have antiseptic properties when airborne and are ideal tonics.

A FEW DROPS

This natural antiseptic is known for the fact that it can be used pure, with direct application to the skin, to heal blemishes, scratches, canker sores, and other minor wounds. One drop on your toothbrush helps fight dental plaque and gives lasting freshness of breath. Purify your office, or any other much-visited place, with this excellent ambient air disinfectant: a few drops in a diffuser will eliminate microbes and miasmas. . . . In the case of chronic fatigue, rub your feet in the morning with one or two drops of tea tree oil. Before you use it for the first time, apply one drop on the hollow of your arm and wait a while to check for any possible (but rare) reaction. Its use is discouraged during pregnancy.

TEA TREE–BASED RECIPES

from Officine Universelle

PURIFYING MASK
FOR BLEMISH- AND BLACKHEAD-
PRONE SKIN

*Whenever your skin loses its balance, treat
yourself to the undeniable virtues of clay
and tea tree.*

Add two teaspoons of tea tree hydrolate
and one teaspoon of hazelnut oil to two
heaping tablespoons of green clay. The
resulting mask is a powerful ally against
unsightly blackheads and other blemishes.
Apply in a thick layer and leave on for
five to seven minutes. You can rehydrate
the outside layer of the mask with a small
sponge if you feel it is drying too quickly.
Delicately rinse off with warm water and
gently pat dry with a soft cloth.

*Perform this ritual once or twice a week
and in the meantime do not try to remove
blemishes and blackheads manually: these
intensive, masochistic attempts do more harm
than good.*

SO LONG, SPOTS!

*Whether your skin is experiencing a full-on
crisis or mere momentary weakness, you're
familiar with these tiny, unsightly outbreaks.
Always keep this fearsome trio of treatment
oils close at hand!*

Fill a small two-ounce jar with a dropper
with macadamia nut oil and add six drops
of tea tree essential oil and six drops
of broadleaved lavender essential oil.
Close the vial tightly and gently shake
the mixture. Massage a small amount of
this disinfecting, drying, and soothing oil
directly onto the blemishes.

FLU-FIGHTING BATH SALTS

*When experiencing fatigue or recovering
from the flu, dive into this reviving and
purifying bath.*

In a glass, add five drops of tea tree
essential oil to one tablespoon of nigella
oil. In a dish, mix seven ounces of coarse
salt with a spoonful of bicarbonate of
soda. Pour the oily mixture onto the
coarse salt and mix with a spoon, then use
this mixture to fill an attractive airtight
container. Prepare this concoction at least
a day in advance, before taking your first
bath enhanced with this treatment salt.

✦ VITELLARIA ✦
(SHEA TREE)

Butter (nuts) — Origin: West Africa

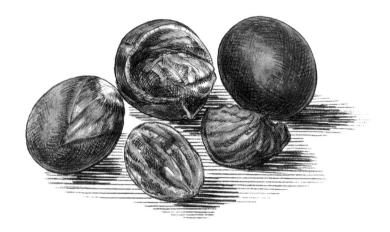

Vitellaria paradoxa

THE AFRICAN

○

Vitellaria paradoxa is a tree that thrives proudly in West and Central Africa. The "belt" formed by its location on the map spans an area characterized by heavy yearly rainfall and a long dry season. The tree is protected by its deep and winding root system, which all the while prevents soil erosion. Its ancient name, *Butyrospermum parkii* ("butter seed"), was an homage to Mungo Park, the famed Scottish explorer, who sailed up the Niger River. His book, *Travels in the Interior of Africa*, described the butter that was extracted from the shea tree's nuts, which was highly prized by the locals. The shea tree yields an abundant and rich oil, used in traditional cooking. Today, due to the risk posed by bush fires, the tree has been included on the list of endangered species by the International Union for Conservation of Nature. Its slow growth and late fructification tend to discourage cultivation.

TEACHINGS FROM TIME IMMEMORIAL

○

In Wolof, its name means "the butter tree," or "life" in the Dyula language. The tree is at the heart of a number of beliefs: it is said that whoever cuts it down will be struck by misfortune. Griots tell a legend about the sacred tree: by the side of his ailing mother, Queen Sogolon Kedjou, the future Mandingo emperor Sundiata Keita solemnly vowed to regain his father's throne. Moved by his nobility of spirit, his mother shared three secrets with him—sacred formulas to be recited to the withered shea tree not far from the maternal hut. "Once you have uttered the first one, the tree will turn green. After the second one, it will bloom, and at the sound of the third, three ripe fruits will fall. Eat these fruits: on all the lands where the shea tree grows, God will ensure your authority," she declared. Sundiata, grief-stricken, went to the tree to recite the magic words. Three ripe nuts fell to the ground. Sundiata ate them and went to bed. By dawn, Sogolon Kedjou had passed away serenely, just as the Sundiata Keita began to reconquer the kingdom.

In his travelogue, the Arab encyclopedist Ibn Fadl Allah-Al'Umari documented the existence of "a tree called kariti, whose fruit is similar to a lime, with a taste that resembles that of the pear, and with a fleshy nut inside. This tender nut is crushed to extract a sort of butter." The roots, leaves, and bark of the shea tree are reputed to heal dysentery, alleviate coughs, and reduce fungal infections. The flowers are melliferous, and the shea tree is a good host for traditional apiculture. The trade and exportation of its butter began in the 19th century with the arrival of Westerners. Locals used it to pay the taxes levied by their colonizers.

ON COLLECTING SHEA BUTTER

◦

The shea tree's nut is made up of 50% fat. Because of its fragility, it is handled gently and dexterously—by women, who have traditionally been in charge of harvesting and processing it. Once washed, dried, crushed, and roasted, the nuts are ground to obtain a thick paste, which is mixed with water and churned. Shea butter is at its best when unrefined and not deodorized. In its natural garb, it has a pale yellow tint, with a light scent that evaporates over time. In spite of its congealed, solid appearance, it remains unctuous, like a balm.

THE BENEFITS

◦

Its nickname, "women's gold," is not unwarranted: the highly concentrated oleic (or omega-9) and stearic fatty acids significantly promote hydration and suppleness of the skin, and reinforce the acid mantle. Vitamin A alleviates patchy skin and accelerates cell turnover, while vitamin E protects against oxidation. Latex and phytosterols improve circulation and absorb UV rays.

"Tall trees grow slowly, but thrust their roots deep in the ground."

AFRICAN WISDOM

HALF A TEASPOON

When it comes to caring for infants, take a cue from the African tradition: massage your baby with some shea butter, warmed and softened between your palms.

Whenever your own skin complains or feels too taut, applying some shea butter to damp skin will restore its balance and nourish that distressed epidermis.

SHEA BUTTER–BASED RECIPES
from Officine Universelle

CLEANSING AND SMOOTHING PASTE

One must learn to relish the nightly ritual of facial cleansing, steering clear of single-use wipes and other such emergency solutions. This gentle balm is suited to all skin types. It gets rid of impurities and relaxes the facial features.

Prepare and sterilize a small flat jar with a screw-on cap. In a ceramic bowl immersed in a bain-marie, melt 2½ teaspoons of shea butter and 2½ teaspoons of beeswax. Remove from the heat and add three tablespoons plus one teaspoon of jojoba oil and a teaspoon of argan oil. Once the preparation has cooled down, add six drops of lavender essential oil and three drops of lemon essential oil. Let it cool down completely and close the jar. Apply the balm by hand, gently massaging it over your face.

Rinse with warm water, pat dry, and finish with an application of rose water. This will keep for a month in a cool, dark place.

VERY, VERY RICH BODY BALM

Does your skin feel lifeless? Time for a major operation! Day in and day out, take the time to massage your whole body with this regenerative balm, to your heart's (and your skin's) content!

Prepare and sterilize a small flat jar with a screw-on cap. In a ceramic bowl immersed in a bain-marie, melt one tablespoon of shea butter and one tablespoon of beeswax. Add a tablespoon of rose hip seed oil and two tablespoons of hemp oil. Allow to cool down, then add three drops of jasmine essential oil and three drops of lemon essential oil.

✦ WHEAT ✦

Oil (grains) — Origin: Middle East

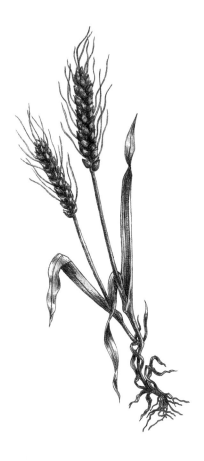

Trictum

BELIEVE YOUR EARS

This cereal, which provides sustenance to much of mankind, is but a modest grass, whose knotty stalk is topped with spiky flowers. *Trictum* – its Latin name – comes in countless varieties, the most common of which (durum wheat, bread wheat, einkorn wheat) have become household names. The earliest types of wheat gathered by man were wild varieties. They were then cultivated, starting in the Neolithic era, in the more irrigated plains of the "fertile crescent" in the Middle East, between the Euphrates and the River Jordan, from east to west. This ancient wheat was "dressed": its bran clung to the grain, from which it was nearly inseparable. Our common wheat was born by crossing emmer with other wild species of wheat. Nowadays, it is cultivated intensively worldwide.

TEACHINGS FROM TIME IMMEMORIAL

o

The sowing and harvesting of wheat sets the tempo for the lives of men. Wheat has a symbolic value across almost all traditions. Superstitions are linked to its cultivation and consumption. It is cited in the Old Testament as well as several other sacred books. At weddings in Ancient Rome, just as in Vedic India, grains of wheat were symbolically poured into the cupped hands of the happy couple. Roman maidens would prepare wheat bran baths to soften their skin. Caterina Sforza, a figure of femininity during the Italian Renaissance, wrote a greatly popular book, *Liber de experimentiis*, in which she compiled beauty and medicinal recipes . . . including a few poisons! Very white skin being in fashion at the time, she recommended the use of wheat bran for its brightening properties. In her *Art of Beauty*, published in 1858, and inspired by a ritual attributed to "the beauties of the Spanish court," Lola Montez recommended it in a recipe for a lotion meant to bring radiance and whiteness to the neck and arms: "Infuse some well-winnowed wheat bran for four hours in some white wine vinegar; add five egg yolks and a pinch of ambergris, and distill this mixture. Seal it hermetically for twelve to fifteen days; you will then be able to use it." On Saint Barbara's Day, December 4, the people of Provence used to plant wheat in three shallow dishes to signal the start of the Christmas season. If, by the day of the Nativity, the wheat had germinated, the harvest would be plentiful.

ON COLLECTING WHEAT

o

Wheat is harvested in summer. The germ is the plant's richest part—full of vitamins, minerals, amino acids, and essential fatty acids. . . . Wheat germ oil is obtained by cold-pressing. It is thick, deep yellow, and redolent of the cereal's warm, round aroma.

THE BENEFITS

o

Wheat germ oil is rich in linoleic acid (omega-6), which protects the skin from external aggressions and efficiently prevents it from drying out. It is second to none in its store of natural active agents: tocopherols, vitamin E . . . all of which are potent antioxidants and help protect the cells from the oxidation caused by free radicals. Vitamin K encourages the coagulation of microvessels: it thus helps to fight rosacea as well as skin redness.

"Let men not be too confident in judging—like he who, in a field, would appraise the wheat before it is ripe."

The Divine Comedy,
DANTE ALIGHIERI

A FEW DROPS

Daily application of wheat germ oil will take good care of mature or irritable skin. Two or three drops of this rich, dense oil will do; each night, massage directly onto the face, taking your time. Wheat germ oil is also a haircare classic: applying it along the length of the hair and leaving it on under a warm towel for a few hours will greatly enhance dry hair.

WHEAT-BASED RECIPES
from Officine Universelle

SARAH BERNHARDT'S BATH

Take a cue from the bath recipe devised by the famed actress: "A kilogram of barley, a pound of rice, a kilo and a half of pulverized lupin seeds, three kilos of bran, one kilo of oat flour, half a pound of lavender." Sarah was not one to take her beauty treatments lightly!

In a large cotton sachet, mix one pound each of wheat bran, barley, and dried lavender. Allow to infuse for fifteen minutes, then step into this milky bath and remain there for about twenty minutes.

FRESH START COMBINATION AND OILY SKIN SCRUB

Our skin is constantly evolving and is liable to switch back and forth between various states. A suitable scrub can help restore its balance. Carefully mix one tablespoon of wheat bran and a teaspoon of honey with one tablespoon of hazelnut oil. Massage this mixture from the face down to the upper neckline area. Remove with a warm cloth and rinse.

ANTIQUE MASK

Round off the cleansing of your skin with this purifying treatment.

Pour two level tablespoons of wheat bran into a bowl, followed by a glass of boiling mineral water. Mix well and allow to infuse for fifteen minutes. Once it has cooled down a bit, pour this paste onto a clean cloth and apply it to the face using the cloth. Leave on for about ten minutes, then remove the mask, gently rubbing your face with the cloth. Rinse with warm water and pat dry with another dry and spotlessly clean cloth.

✦ WITCH HAZEL ✦

Leaves and bark, hydrolate — Origin: North America

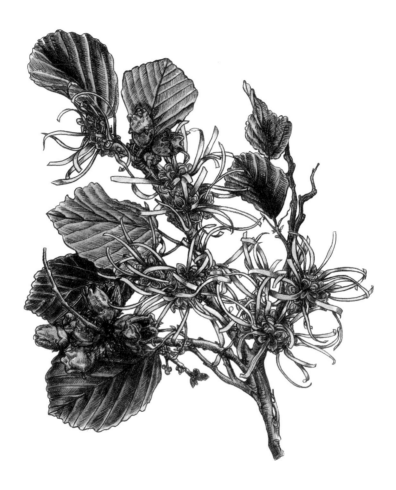

Hamamelis virginiana

THE DEVIL'S COFFEE

○

Hamamelis virginiana is a hardy shrub which in winter adorns itself with small, pale yellow flowers, once its fuzzy leaves have fallen. Hailing from North America, it has now spread to Europe.

TEACHINGS FROM TIME IMMEMORIAL

○

Amerindians used to see witch hazel as a magical plant with a unique status in nature: in defiance of the natural rhythm of the seasons, it blossoms in winter. The Osage used its bark to heal ulcers, the

Pottawatomi heated its twigs on coals in their sweat lodges to relax aching muscles, and the Iroquois used it as a decoction against dysentery, colds, and coughs. Its English name refers to the flexibility of its branches, which are used to craft divining rods for finding springs or mineral lodes. The Mohegan reportedly demonstrated this power to the earliest European settlers. Described in 1736 by the American botanist John Bartram, founder of the first botanical garden in New England, witch hazel was sent to Europe sometime around 1750. In 1935, in his *Flore Laurentienne*, an inventory of the flora of the Saint Lawrence River valley, Brother Marie-Victorin mentioned that witch hazel was commonly used in Quebec to enrich shaving lotions and soften the skin. It is found in the patented formulas of beauty products and miracle creams that incorporate witch hazel bark. Steam distillation of dormant branches harvested in the spring, augmented with alcohol, creates the famed "Witch Hazel Water," a skin tonic which was highly popular at the beginning of the last century in Europe and the United States.

ON PREPARING WITCH HAZEL

Witch hazel leaves are harvested in summer and put out to dry as quickly as possible. The hydrolate derived from the steam distillation of these flowers smells like freshly cut hay.

THE BENEFITS

With its high concentration of tannins, witch hazel is known for its astringent properties and its ability to stimulate venous circulation. The rutin it contains has phlebotonic properties. Its significant bioflavonoid content supports the walls of blood vessels—it is said to be "vasoconstructive."

A FEW DROPS

Used as a lotion in the morning and at night, witch hazel hydrolate is a panacea for sensitive, redness-prone skin. For combination and oily skin types, it will round off the cleansing process, tightening the pores. Cold compresses soaked in hydrolate and applied below the eyes will reawaken them and minimize bags. The hydrolate is also used in summer to soothe mosquito bites.

WITCH HAZEL–BASED RECIPES

from Officine Universelle

HAPPY MORNING AFTER

Last night's party was a blast, but now you need to smooth out your appearance and revive your complexion.

Pour one tablespoon of witch hazel hydrolate into a bowl, and add a tablespoon of aloe vera gel and a small teaspoon of freshly shelled and ground almonds. Massage this mask on the face like a scrub, then leave on for ten minutes. Rinse with warm water and dry gently.

REFRESHING AND DEODORIZING LOTION

Keeping your body odor to yourself is an excellent resolution: this lotion is as natural as it is effective.

Using a bamboo whisk, mix seven tablespoons of witch hazel hydrolate with two tablespoons of vegetal glycerin, about six drops of palmarosa essential oil, and about six drops of green mandarin essential oil. Using a soaked cotton pad, rub this lotion under your armpits, on your bosom, and on the nape of your neck.

PRETTY LEG WRAP

Enhance your summer legwork with this wrap and gently lighten your diet, starting by removing sugar and white bread.

Dilute ten tablespoons of green clay in ¾ cup plus one tablespoon of witch hazel hydrolate. Apply this in a thick layer from the top of the thigh to the knee, down to the back of the calf if necessary. Remain standing peacefully in the bathroom, a good book in hand, for about ten minutes. In the shower, rinse with warm and then cold water, working your way up from the big toe to the inside of the knee to the top of the thigh, then rinse the outside of the leg. Focus on the hollow behind the knee in order to stimulate lymphatic circulation.

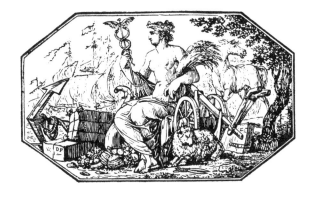

RECIPE INDEX

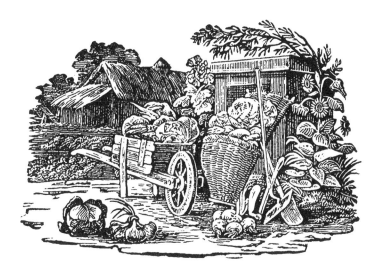

WHO ARE YOU?

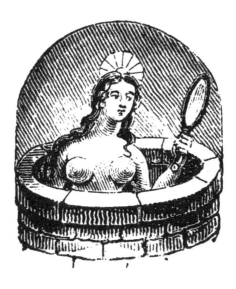

Taking care of yourself is a personal journey, punctuated by countless experiences and discoveries. Getting intimately acquainted with yourself and knowing how to satisfy your own needs so as to feel beautiful and good leads to self-enrichment.

Beauty is not something that should be left to the professionals; there is no single way to take care of yourself, but your way is the best way.

Here is some starting advice to guide your first steps and adapt your skincare routine to your skin type. The latter becomes rather settled during adulthood, yet your skin may experience variations as it becomes dehydrated or sensitive.

What do you see when you look at yourself in a magnifying mirror?

Your face gives off a certain radiance. Your skin is not a troublemaker; it is soft to the touch; it looks even and has a fine, tight grain, an absence of shine, and a comfortable feel. This is normal skin.

Your matte, fine-textured skin often feels tight, but it has a fine, good-looking grain. When it is giving you a hard time, it can have a rough or cracked texture to the touch — so-called crocodile skin syndrome. Yours is dry skin.

You have a dreary air and a dull complexion. You experience a persistent sense of discomfort and tightness;

sometimes your eyebrows or the sides of your nose tend to flake. Yours is dehydrated skin.

Your face is slightly shiny; the skin of your forehead and nose is oilier than that of your cheeks. Your pores appear larger on the T-zone, where the sweat glands are more heavily concentrated. Your cheeks are more sensitive and often display some redness after showering. Yours is combination skin.

Your face is shiny. Your skin grain is coarser and more irregular; you are prone to experiencing blemishes and blackheads; your pores are visible. Yours is oily skin.

Your skin is very prone to redness as well as itches, irritations, and unusual allergies. Yours is sensitive skin.

If in doubt, try the well-known tissue paper test. After cleansing and drying your face, wait for about thirty minutes and cut two strips of tissue paper, about one and a half inches wide. Apply the first one to your T-zone (forehead, nose, and chin) and the other to a temple and a cheek. Keep those in place for two minutes, without rubbing the skin.

If both strips show numerous stains, your skin is probably oily.

If only the strip that was applied to your T-zone is stained, you have combination skin.

If both strips show few stains, your skin is normal.

If neither of the strips is stained at all, you have dry skin.

Pay attention to the evolution of your skin on a day-to-day basis or in periods of seasonal change. You will notice it evolves and requires more attention during stressful times or periods of intense fatigue. When you are on vacation, you will forget all about it. Adapt your regimen to these variations, and when your usual routine no longer works, adjust it by trusting your instincts and your sensations. Your skin is talking to you: listen to it.

What do you see when you look at yourself in a magnifying mirror?

LIST OF CONCERNS

A nonexhaustive list of some mind, skin, and hair concerns.

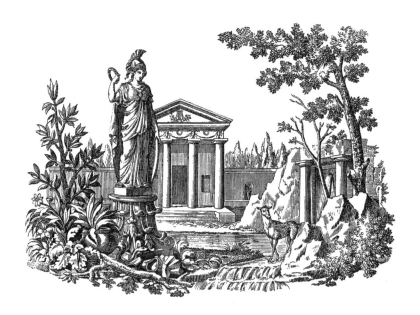

MIND CONCERNS

◦

MOOD ENHANCER
Geranium, jasmine, mint, rose, sake.

TEMPER-SOOTHING
Chamomile, corn poppy, lavender, rosemary.

SKIN CONCERNS

◦

AGE BEAUTIFULLY
Açaí, amla, argan, borage, camellia, evening primrose, ginkgo biloba, grape, hibiscus, Inca Inchi, lily, perilla, pomegranate, pear, rose, sake.

BALANCING
Grape, jojoba, Kalahari melon.

BLEMISH-PRONE SKIN
Argan, clays, copaiba, geranium, honey, nigella, rosemary, tea tree.

BRIGHTENING COMPLEXION
Apricot, azuki, buriti, corn poppy, cornflower, iris, lotus, pearl, rose, seaweeds.

SOOTHING AND HEALING PROPERTIES
Arnica, clays, copaiba, lavender, marigold, nigella, oats, tamanu.

CELLULITE
Andiroba, chaulmoogra, loofah.

CIRCULATION BOOSTER
Andiroba, daisy, lemon, marula, olive, tea, vitellaria.

DRY SKIN

Açaí, argan, avocado, cocoa, hemp, honey, kukui, mongongo, olive, raspberry, sesame, sweet almond, vitellaria.

EXHAUSTED SKIN

Açaí, baobab, *Centella asiatica*, rice, hemp, rosemary, salt.

FIGHTING POLLUTION
AND EXTERNAL AGGRESSIONS

Rice, sea buckthorn, wheat.

ITCHINESS

Borage, chaulmoogra, kukui, sweet almond.

LIP AND MOUTH CARE

Castor seed, coconut, iris, honey, miswak.

PORE TIGHTENING

Geranium, marula, rose, witch hazel.

REDNESS

Hemp, Inca Inchi, pomegranate, raspberry, tamanu, wheat, witch hazel.

SENSITIVE AND REACTIVE SKIN

Aloe vera, borage, marigold, oats, peony, St. John's wort.

SLOWING BODY HAIR REGROWTH

Nut grass.

STRETCHMARKS

Avocado, cocoa, tamanu.

SUNBURN

Aloe vera, mint, St. John's wort.

SUNSPOTS

Chaulmoogra, lily.

TIRED AND PUFFY EYES

Chamomile, cornflower, jasmine, tamanu, tea, witch hazel.

HAIR CONCERNS

BRIGHTENING ACTION FOR
NORMAL HAIR

Camellia, chamomile, jojoba, wheat.

DANDRUFF

Neem.

DRY HAIR

Andiroba, avocado, Brazil nut, coconut, olive.

FINE HAIR

Passion fruit, rose.

FRIZZY HAIR

Andiroba, baobab.

GRAY HAIR

Amla.

HAIR IN DISTRESS

Castor seed, centella, chamomile.

HAIR LOSS

Castor seed, pracaxi, sapote.

IRRITATED SCALP

Aloe vera, clays, pracaxi, peony, sesame.

OILY HAIR

Neem, jojoba.

STIMULATE REGROWTH

Hibiscus, passion fruit, sapote.

TABLE
OF
TREATMENTS

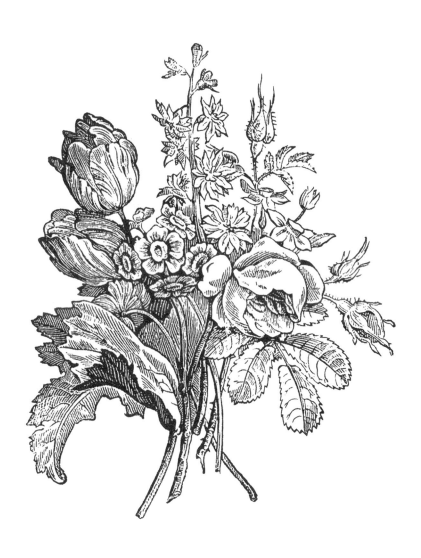

FACE

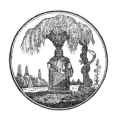

MOISTURIZING

Apricot Facial radiance ointment

Argan Antioxidant healing facial serum

Fresh complexion EVENING PRIMROSE treatment oil

Hemp Balancing oil

Subsolar PEONY oil

Phaeacia facial St. John's wort oil

Hananotsuyu, or flower dew (SESAME)

Miracle PRACAXI treatment for patchy hands and necklines

Miracle soothing BORAGE fluid for the face and neckline

Post-sun BURITI emergency treatment

White LILY youth elixir

Balance-restoring Kalahari melon facial

"Three continents, three cures" oil (PERILLA)

Potent antiaging PRICKLY PEAR serum

Rose Radiant facial boost

Rose Bracing facial fluid

Anti-redness SEA BUCKTHORN youth serum

Sea buckthorn subsolar oil

CLEANSING

Açaí makeup remover for all occasions

Purifying CLAY facial mask

Universal NIGELLA purifying mask

Gentle SWEET ALMOND exfoliant for the face and lips

Purifying, brightening TAMANU mask for the face and neckline

Cleansing and smoothing VITELLARIA paste

Antique WHEAT mask

Radiant beauty softening mask (BEE)

Gentlest facial CAMELLIA cleansing mask

Extra-purifying KALAHARI MELON scrub

Gentle RASPBERRY seed oil facial exfoliant

Great Pacific KUKUI facial cleanse

Raspberry facial cleansing milk

Deep-cleaning SAKE-based facial lotion

Dream night LAVENDER pillow

At summer's end, a LILY complexion

Rice belle

Go green TEA

Unctuous, COCOA restorative balm

GINKGO balancing cleansing paste

Purifying, makeup-removing SESAME oil

TONING

Instant COCONUT tone-brightening mask

Toning CORNFLOWER facial lotion

Toning DAISY treatment for the face, neck, and neckline area

"Sunday complexion" JASMINE mask

Sacred LOTUS enlightening mask

Pink SAKE and PERILLA lotion

Instant beauty POMEGRANATE recovery mask

Alabaster complexion (RICE)

"Bright eyes and clear skin" ROSE treatment

The new Queen of Hungary's water (ROSEMARY)

Purifying MINT mist

TEA Mizudashi lotion

CALMING

Raspberry seed oil–based arnica macerate

Aloe vera SOS sun balm

The thousand-virtue MARIGOLD ointment

Brightening, anti-redness PASSION FRUIT facial treatment

Soothing and restorative PEONY mask

Anti-rosacea TAMANU facial oil

Beautifying BURITI body treatment for sun-kissed skin

Soothing CENTELLA ASIATICA balm for damaged and irritated skin

Anti-rosacea INCA INCHI serum

Softening PRICKLY PEAR pulp mask

Help—lifesaving AÇAÍ mask for skin in need

You own ST. JOHN'S WORT macerate

BALANCING

Apricot and ROSE purifying and stimulating mask

ARGAN treatment mask for the face and chest

Azuki Balancing facial mask

Smoothing, decongesting CORNFLOWER mask

GINKGO-based eternal beauty mask

High-radiance GRAPE mask

Facial MARULA balancing treatment

Great aura INCA INCHI mask

Brightening and balancing IRIS facial mask

Happy morning after (WITCH HAZEL)

Fresh start WHEAT combination and oily skin scrub

BLEMISHES

ANDIROBA soothing anti-mosquito balm

"Farewell blemishes" COPAIBA balm

Calming GERANIUM lotion for blemish-prone skin

So long, spots! (TEA TREE)

SOS ointment for acne (BEE)

Purifying facial LAVENDER steam bath

Purifying TEA TREE mask for blemish- and blackhead-prone skin

EYES & LIPS

○

Eyebrow growth CASTOR SEED serum

"Kiss me" CASTOR SEED balm

Soothing CHAMOMILE treatment for teething infants

Intense KOHL

Bye bye blues (MINT)

SALT toothpaste

SESAME gandoush

OLIVE pretty gums

HAIR

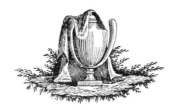

CLEANSING

Argan oil-enhanced shampoo

Softest AZUKI cleanser for a stressed scalp

Purple SEAWEED fortifying shampoo

Radiance-restoring BURITI shampoo for dull, lifeless hair

Stimulating anti-hair loss CENTELLA ASIATICA shampoo for tired hair

Purifying JOJOBA mask for irritated scalps

HYDRATING

Special AÇAÍ serum for split ends

Stimulating and nourishing AMLA preshampoo fluid for dark hair

Avocado oil-based nourishing hair mask

Fiery HIBISCUS treatment for radiant red hair

Anti-dry tips MONGONGO hair mask

Thirst-quenching OATS mask for dry hair

Reviving BAOBAB mask for coarse hair

Nourishing and straightening CAMELLIA hair-rinsing lotion

Island hair mask (KUKUI)

SHINE

Hydrating HIBISCUS hair lotion for copper-colored volume

The great blond MARIGOLD rinsing water

Passion FRUIT treatment for perennially beautiful hair

Beautiful shoreline rinse (SEAWEEDS)

Hananotsuyu, or flower dew (SESAME)

Strength and shine hair balm (BEE)

LEMON Shine water ROSE VINEGAR

FORTIFYING

Anti-hair loss ALOE VERA hydrating mask

Fast-growth AMLA hair fortifier

Avocado pulp-based fortifying hair mask

Fortifying and stimulating NIGELLA oil for the hair

Preserving, anti-hair loss PRACAXI serum

Fortifying oil for the hair and scalp (SWEET ALMOND)

Fortifying BRAZIL NUT oil bath for the hair

Fortifying COCOA mask for strong hair

SAPOTE strong hair mask

ATTITUDE
○

SALT beach hair spray

HAIR ISSUES
○

Dandruff emergency oily and irritated scalp (NEEM)

SAKE purifying, anti-dandruff lotion for the scalp

Down with lice! (NEEM)

BODY

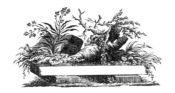

HYDRATING

SOS ALOE VERA sun balm

Raspberry seed oil–based ARNICA macerate

BAOBAB anti–stretch mark oil

Soothing CENTELLA ASIATICA balm for damaged and irritated skin

Anti-itch CHAULMOOGRA balm

The DAISY odalisque's oil—"Down with hairs and fat dimples!"

Revitalizing HEMP body oil

The thousand-virtue MARIGOLD ointment

Egyptian SESAME oil

Anti–stretch mark TAMANU serum

Beautifying body BURITI treatment for sun-kissed skin

TREATMENT

COCOA and CYPRESS slimming treatment

Eczema emergency CENTELLA ASIATICA poultice

RHASSOUL and HONEY body wrap

COCONUT and SUGAR body scrub

Toning DAISY treatment for the face, neck, and neckline area

GINKGO BILOBA heavy leg treatment

Softest LEMON body wrap

Sunny day MARULA body treatment

MENTHOL body scrub

Reviving, purifying SAKE rubdown for the body and neckline area

Summer body stimulating SALT scrub

Slimming green TEA body scrub

Pretty leg WITCH HAZEL wrap

Refreshing and deodorizing WITCH HAZEL lotion

BATH

BORAGE flower beauty bath

Temper-soothing CHAMOMILE bath

Remineralizing CLAY bath

IRIS purifying bath

JASMINE Bridal bath

"Mood-altering" LAVENDER bath

Relaxing aromatic MINT bath

Irritation-soothing
OAT bath

Comforting PEONY bath

RICE vinegar summer bath

Deep-sea bath (SEAWEEDS)

Green TEA bath salt
Flu-fighting TEA TREE
bath salts

Sarah Bernhardt's WHEAT
bath

Quick! My salts! (GERANIUM)

MASSAGE
ο

Draning ANDIROBA massage
oil

Relaxing COPAIBA massage
after exercise

Soothing GERANIUM
self-massage

"Follow me" JASMINE
massage oil

Draining and reviving
JOJOBA massage oil

OLIVE massage scrub

HANDS & FEET
ο

Purifying hand and foot
ALUM STONE scrub

Clarifying, fortifying
CHAMOMILE nail bath

Anti-callus COPAIBA serum

Queenly feet (LEMON)

Miracle PRACAXI treatment
for patchy hands

Light-footed ROSEMARY
bath

Spectacular elbow,
hand, and foot BRAZIL
NUT scrub

BODY HAIR
MAINTENANCE
ο

The DAISY odalisque's
oil — "Down with hairs and
fat dimples!"

Sugar-LEMON waxing paste

OLIVE shaving oil

INDEX

A FEW
BEAUTY ESSENTIALS
AT YOUR SERVICE

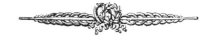

Grab your needles and scissors.

Natural beauty can be improved upon through the use of small bags that come in very handy for a number of recipes.

Select a bleached or raw organic cotton fabric to create these versatile sachets, which will make it easier to enjoy the full benefits of clays, powders, and herbs.

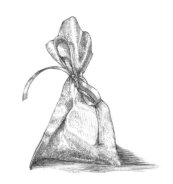

THE SMALL
FACIAL CLEANSING SACHET
(2 x 2¼ inches)

The chosen fabric must be very thin, allowing the contents to be absorbed by your skin. We recommend its use with rice bran as well as iris, rose, lavender, peony, lotus, and ginkgo biloba powder. Humidify the sachet with some mineral water and apply delicately to the face.

After use, hang on a hook and allow to dry in the open air—this will enable you to use it a second time before you have to empty and wash it.

THE MEDIUM-SIZED BAG
(4 x 3½ inches)

Designed for body exfoliation, or for the soapless cleansing of the most delicate skin types. It is ideal for clays, oats, tea, and wheat. Humidify the bag and rub it over your body.

After use, hang on a hook and allow to dry in the open air—this will enable you to use it a second time before you have to empty and wash it.

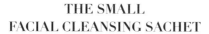

THIS ALL-PURPOSE BAG
(6 x 8¼ inches)

An oversized version of a tea bag, this allows you to create your own aromatic baths by blending flower petals, cereals, and fragrant herbs while avoiding any collateral damage to your bathtub.

It is essential when using borage, rosemary, lavender, mint, geranium, jasmine, olive tree leaves, St. John's wort, seaweeds, and chamomile.

Dive into your warm bath as soon as it is half full so as to benefit from all of those lovely fragrances.

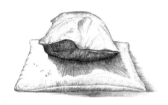

MAKURA, THE BUCKWHEAT HULL PILLOW
(14 x 19½ inches)

To achieve beauty, beauty sleep is a must. In Japan, where they are known as *sobakawa*, dried buckwheat hulls are used to fill firm-to-the-touch pillows that provide support for the neck and relax the upper spine.

Buckwheat helps regulate body temperature.

Fill the pillowcase to your liking. It must be left out in the sun regularly and does not tolerate humidity.

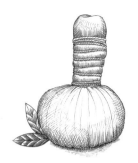

THAI POUCH
(8½ x 11½ inches)

This Thai massage tool enables you to relax painful areas or to massage your loved ones.

In a rather firm piece of cotton fabric, cut out a rectangle, 8½ by 11½ inches in size. Fill it with a blend of seeds, dried herbs, and dampened and dried clay and grind the whole thing to a powder. Using the fabric, fashion this into a tight ball, tie a small knot at the base, and twist the rest of the fabric into a tight handle (use the string to keep it together, working your way from the base of the handle to the top). You should be left with a ball topped by a handle, giving you an easy grasp.

After slightly humidifying this bundle, steam it for a minute to warm it up and check its temperature before applying to your face or body for a relaxing massage.

ACKNOWLEDGMENTS

We are extremely grateful to all the visitors of our Officine on rue Bonaparte who, standing at our counter, have shared with us their beauty stories, their childhood and bathroom memories, and above all how they take care of themselves. They are an invaluable source of inspiration and information.

Beauty is a family affair, and both of us were lucky enough to be well-schooled on that count. What would we be without the doting care that was bestowed upon us? Without this contagious enthusiasm that ran in our families? Without them telling us about their latest cosmetic adventures? Scherazade, Adam, and Noor are now the docile guinea pigs of our own experiments. We thank them tenderly.

We are also very grateful to the staff of L'Officine Universelle Buly, who work wonders on a daily basis and got generously involved in the research, fact-checking, and countless experiments required to test the enclosed recipes, and in particular: Berenice Clerc, Julie Parage, Nedjma Amrani, Emiko Oguri, Sofia Barrouche, Myriam Garcette, Sarah de Mavaleix, and Jana Hoppe.

This Atlas is highly indebted to the knowledge of our suppliers and to the passion with which they tell the story of their "products." We are proud to offer them and to share what they have taught us. Special thanks go to Carole Tawema, Khalid Jaafria, the El-Hedda sisters, Izabel Barros, and Mitsuji Inamura.

Conceiving, writing, and perfecting this Atlas has been a fascinating, joyful, and collegial experience. A thousand thanks go to Stéphanie Hussonnois-Bouhayati, who generously puts her quill and quickness of spirit at the service of L'Officine and who has been with us on this project from the start; to Susanna Lea, Kerry Glencorse, and Emmanuelle Hardouin, who enjoyed the book to the point of modifying their beauty routines (!); to Lizzy Gray and her whole team for their enthusiasm and patience; to Marie Levi for the layout and her sense of detail; to Julien Guieu for translating our prose with composure and wit; and to Pierre and Marie-Cécile de Taillac for their always pertinent advice.

MERCI

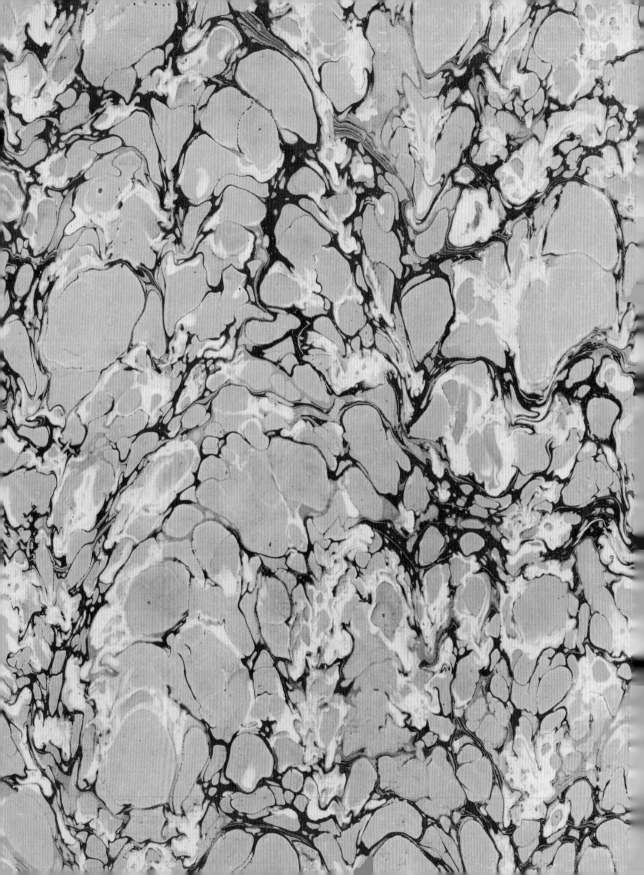